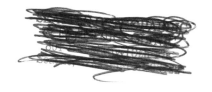

Spine

Prolotherapy in the Lumbar Spine and Pelvis

Editor:

Thomas A. Dorman, MD
Private Practice
San Luis Obispo, California

Volume 9/Number 2
HANLEY & BELFUS, INC.

May 1995
Philadelphia

STATE OF THE ART REVIEWS

Publisher: HANLEY & BELFUS, INC.
210 South 13th Street
Philadelphia, PA 19107
(215) 546-4995
Fax (215) 790-9330

SPINE: State of the Art Reviews   **(ISSN 0887-9869)**
Volume 9, Number 2   **(ISBN 1-56053-187-8)**

Authorization to photocopy items for internal or personal use, or the internal or personal use
of specific clients, is granted by Hanley & Belfus, Inc. for libraries and other users regis-
tered with the Copyright Clearance Center (CCC) Transaction Reporting Service, provided
that the base fee of $1.00 per copy plus $0.25 per page is paid directly to the CCC, 21
Congress St., Salem, MA 01970. Identify this publication by including with your payment the
fee code, 0887-9869/95 $1.00 + .25.

SPINE: State of the Art Reviews is published triannually (three times per year) by Hanley &
Belfus, Inc., 210 South 13th Street, Philadelphia, Pennsylvania 19107.

POSTMASTER: Send address changes to SPINE: State of the Art Reviews, Hanley & Belfus,
Inc., 210 South 13th Street, Philadelphia, PA 19107.

SPINE: State of the Art Reviews
Vol. 9, No. 2, 1995

PROLOTHERAPY IN THE LUMBAR SPINE
AND PELVIS
Thomas A. Dorman, MD, Editor

CONTENTS

> Dr. Mooney provides a personal account of how he came to believe in prolotherapy for the treatment of patients with chronic pain in the back and pelvis. It was not until he witnessed prolotherapy's benefits in patients in whom the standard orthopedic surgical approach had failed that he became convinced of its usefulness.

> This overview of the many new ideas contained in this volume describes the role of the pelvis and sacroiliac joints in human walking, including the view that the pelvis functions as a mechanically unique link in the transfer of the forces between the legs and trunk.

> Dr. Dorman discusses the context of orthopedic medicine within the larger realm of allopathic medicine. Readers are acquainted with concepts such as asymlocation of the pelvis, tensegrity, referred pain, posain, and nulliness. A brief history of healing techniques is presented, beginning with Hippocrates' use of searing to stabilize the shoulders of the warriors of Sparta.

> Recent advances in understanding the structure and innervation of the lumbosacral region are examined. The author explains that the tissues of the lumbosacral connection receive a nerve supply capable of sustaining a prolonged inflammatory response, thus contributing to the progressive breakdown of function in the back.

The Importance of Soft Tissues for Structural Support of the Body 357
Stephen M. Levin

Various structural models are explored in an attempt to identify constructs that are analogous to biologic modeling. Since only trusses are inherently stable with freely moving hinges, the author concludes that vertebrates with flexible joints must be constructed as trusses.

Elastic Energy in the Pelvis 365
Thomas A. Dorman

This chapter suggests that ligaments and fasciae in the pelvis store elastic energy and that dysfunction of the pelvic mechanism is often a source of back pain. The clinical diagnosis and practical therapeutics by orthopedic medical means are discussed, and increased efficiency in walking after treatment with prolotherapy is demonstrated.

The Sacrum in Three-Dimensional Space 381
Stephen M. Levin

Based on the idea that biologic structures must obey all the rules of physics and mechanics, a new model for sacral mechanics is proposed that accounts for both the statics and dynamics of the sacrum in vertebrates. The model suggests that the sacrum, as the hub of a tension network, provides stability during walking.

Lower Extremity Mechanics and Their Effect on Lumbosacral Function 389
Howard J. Dananberg

A framework is given for understanding the mechanics of human gait and the intricate interrelationships of the structures of the lower limbs. The author asserts that recognition that degenerative joint disease, disk herniation, and myogenic pain may result from a gait-related process is essential in order to treat patients effectively.

Self-Locking of the Sacroiliac Articulation 407
Thomas A. Dorman and Andry Vleeming

Taking a reductionist point of view, the authors review recent research and propose that the human sacroiliac joint functions as a key element in the pelvis. The proposal is supported by the introduction of new concepts, such as force closure and form closure, the transfer of antigravitational and elastic energy, and the integrated function of muscles, ligaments, and fasciae.

Biomechanical Modeling of Sacroiliac Joint Stability in Different Postures 419
C. J. Snijders, A. Vleeming, R. Stoeckart, J. M. A. Mens, G. J. Kleinrensink

This chapter discusses the transfer of load from the spine to the innominate bones and legs, with special attention to the stability of the sacroiliac joints. A biomechanical model that begins with identification of the mechanical vulnerability of the sacroiliac joints is described. Electromyographic findings and mechanical solutions to protect the joints against dislocation that validate the underlying model are presented.

The Slipping Clutch Syndrome 433
Thomas A. Dorman

> When patients who were receiving prolotherapy to the posterior sacroiliac liga-
> ments began expressing gratitude that their episodic falling had been cured, the
> author made a connection between episodic falling and function of the sacroiliac
> joint. This and other clinical observations led him to define "the slipping clutch
> syndrome," the acceptance of which hinges on the recognition of various principles
> in orthopedic medicine.

Imaging Mechanical Dysfunctions of the Spine 437
Thomas H. Ravin

> This well-illustrated chapter seeks to bridge the gap that prevents radiologists from
> being able to identify simple somatic joint dysfunctions with their hands and clini-
> cians from being able to identify the presence of osteitis condenses illi on plain
> film.

Gravitational Stress, Musculoligamentous Strain, and Postural
Alignment 463
Michael L. Kuchera

> Gravitational force, a constant and underestimated stressor of the somatic system,
> is discussed with regard to its effect on muscle, ligaments, other fasciae, and the re-
> lationship of each to posture and skeletal alignment. Radiographic findings and
> treatment protocols are detailed.

Functional Biomechanics and Management of Pathomechanics
of the Sacroiliac Joints. 491
Richard L. DonTigny

> The author describes the function of the sacroiliac joints; a specific, measurable,
> reversible, biomechanical dysfunction of the joint; and ways to evaluate and
> manage this dysfunction, including the use of the passive straight-leg raising test,
> mobilization techniques, corrective exercises, various modalities, and invasive
> procedures.

Refurbishing Ligaments with Prolotherapy 509
Thomas A. Dorman

> A range of aspects of prolotherapy are succinctly covered here—from a philosoph-
> ical introduction, to a discussion of the endpoints of healing; from description of
> the evidence of a proliferant's effect, to the applicability of Wolff's law.

Index 517

CONTRIBUTORS

Howard J. Dananberg, DPM, FACFAOM
Bedford Podiatry Group, The Walking Clinic, Bedford, New Hampshire; podiatry staff, Catholic Medical Center, Elliot Hospital, Manchester, New Hampshire

Richard L. DonTigny, PT
DonTigny Physical Therapy, Havre, Montana

Thomas A. Dorman, MB, ChB, MRCP(UK), FRCP(C)
Private Practice, San Luis Obispo, California

G. J. Kleinrensink, MSc
Assistant Professor, Department of Anatomy, Erasmus University, Rotterdam, The Netherlands

Michael L. Kuchera, DO, FAAO
Professor and Chairman, Department of Osteopathic Manipulative Medicine, Kirksville College of Osteopathic Medicine, Kirksville, Missouri

Stephen M. Levin, MD
Director, Potomac Back Center, Vienna, Virginia

Johannes Martinus Adrianus Mens, MD
Assistant Professor, Department of Rehabilitation Medicine, Erasmus University, Rotterdam, The Netherlands

Vert Mooney, MD
Professor of Orthopedic Surgery, Department of Orthopedic Surgery, University of California, San Diego, California

Thomas H. Ravin, MD
Private Practice, Denver, Colorado

Christiaan J. Snijders, PhD
Professor, Department Head, Department of Biomedical Physics and Technology, Faculty of Medicine and Allied Health Sciences, Erasmus University, Rotterdam, The Netherlands

Rob Stoeckart, PhD
Senior Lecturer, Department of Anatomy, Erasmus University, Rotterdam, The Netherlands

Andry Vleeming, PhD
Associate Professor, Department of Anatomy, Erasmus University, Rotterdam, The Netherlands

Frank H. Willard, PhD
Associate Professor of Anatomy, Department of Anatomy, University of New England, Biddeford, Maine; European School of Osteopathy, Maidstone, Kent, England

PREFACE

This issue of Spine: State of the Art Reviews brings together an interdisciplinary approach to the human pelvis. Prolotherapy, a form of injection therapy for the management of ligament relaxation, is the leitmotif.

Between the covers of this issue are the cooperative writings of a few university-based researchers and a number of clinicians. This relationship is as it should be in the advancement of a clinical science. The reader will find differences in emphasis and opinion among the contributors. The editor has made no attempt to gloss them over. It is through the dialectic of discussion that further advances will come.

The human pelvis has certain characteristics that differentiate it from that of nonbiped mammals. These unique features have been shown recently to have great clinical significance. The chapter by Vleeming and Dorman elucidates it as a gearbox (transducer) for the transfer of the forces of locomotion. The connective tissue of our bodies, predominantly ligamentous, is an organ in itself, even though it is diffusely distributed; the fascia is continuous. Willard's illustrations make this point elegantly. The function of this organ is also continuous, diffuse, and essential for the storage and release of elastic energy in locomotion. The fascial organ functions as a *tensegrity* model. Levin's chapters explain this new concept. In bipedal walking an exception to the diffuse distribution of force occurs in the sacroiliac articulation with walking. The concepts of force closure and self-bracing, which were developed by Vleeming, Snijders, and their team, explain the unique function of this articulation. The clinical counterpart, dysfunction, is the subject of several other chapters. The reader will find a new way for the mobilization of the pelvis in DonTigny's chapter and an overview of an osteopathic approach by Kuchera, with an emphasis on the role of gravity. The imaging counterparts can be found in Ravin's chapter. Since the lower limb is integral to locomotion, fascial-ligamentous failure often involves the whole lower section of a person's body. Dananberg's chapter on the lower limb introduces the additional concept, in foot dysfunction, of the functional hallux limitus.

It is anticipated that this issue will stimulate the already burgeoning interest in the fascial-ligamentous organ and its importance, not only in back pain but in sprains that lead to chronic disability from all the moving parts of the body. Clinicians wishing to learn the use of prolotherapy will need to hone their diagnostic skills in orthopedic medicine. One organization with which to start this process is the American Association of Orthopaedic Medicine.[1]

THOMAS DORMAN, MD
GUEST EDITOR

---

1 The American Association of Orthopaedic Medicine is located at 435 North Michigan Ave., Suite 1717, Chicago IL 60611-4067. Phone: (800) 992-2063.

VERT MOONEY, MD

PROLOTHERAPY IN THE SPINE AND PELVIS: AN INTRODUCTION

From the UCSD OrthoMed Center
Department of Orthopedics
University of California, San Diego
La Jolla, California

Reprint requests to:
Vert Mooney, MD
Professor of Orthopedics
UCSD OrthoMed Center
4150 Regents Park Row
Suite 300
La Jolla, CA 92037

This introduction will take the form of a somewhat personal account of my own education about the world of soft tissue medicine. Soft tissue medicine has been described as orthopedic medicine. It is the world of evaluation to find weak ligaments and inflamed fascial attachments. It is a conceptual framework that recognizes the interconnection of posture, gait, and balance. It is to the credit of the publishers of this series, Spine: State of the Art Reviews, that they will make this fascinating world visible to those interested in understanding the spine. It is also to the credit of Dr. Tom Dorman, editor of this volume, who has made so many contributions to this area.

My background in spinal care was completely traditional and, thus, very narrow. I, like every resident orthopedic surgeon in training, dreaded the low back clinic: the land of assumed psychological cripples presenting with unknowable disease—an endless series of returning patients who had had treatments that did not work. The treatments, whether surgical or pharmacologic, seemed to have no effect on a disease process that was disabling to manual workers, housewives, and even bank executives who couldn't golf appropriately. It was clear that we did not understand many of the real causes of back pain.

As my career progressed, I became more sensitive than the average orthopedic surgeon to rehabilitation issues. I attribute this to my training at Rancho Los Amigos Hospital, a large rehabilitation hospital in the Los Angeles area. The training offered me an unusual experience that was verified by the 600 or so orthopedic residents who had some training there. There was much to be learned from the evaluation of our allied health colleagues in physical and occupation therapy. Traditional physical examination of orthopedic trainees did not offer an appropriate sense for the inadequacy of muscle and fascial function. Certainly we could evaluate a neurologic deficit, but the majority of chronic musculoskeletal problems had additional causes of dysfunction not explained by neuromotor-controlled barriers. Although the standard medical model provided by the marvelous Netter anatomic drawings indicated that all of the problems had been corrected, many people did not get better. The role of sensitive palpation for evaluation and manual therapy for treatment was clarified by these therapists.

As I progressed into practice, I found that people were paying me to determine the causes of vague and recurrent problems still unexplained by the standard orthopedic surgical models. The failures to improve were blamed on their own psychological inadequacies.

I eventually became chairman of an orthopedic training program and served as president of the Orthopedic Chairman's Association. I was involved with tasks such as establishing the body of knowledge appropriate for orthopedic surgeons, developing tests, and monitoring tests. I felt comfortable that I knew what an orthopedic surgeon should know. Nonetheless, important topics went uncovered. People still had confusing chronic musculoskeletal problems, unresolved by standard exercise programs or the ever-present steroid injections. Although steroid injections were valuable, they often did not provide a persistent cure to the inflammatory lesion being treated. And we surely did not know where to operate on these patients.

As the techniques of surgery improved in the world of orthopedic care, more and more problems became solvable by the greatly improved equipment and understanding available to us by improved diagnostic studies. Fractures that once caused months of medical care and resulted in prolonged and sometimes permanent disability were now treated with a few hours of expert surgery using marvelously designed equipment. The arthroscope cured many structural abnormalities in a very benign way. Access became available to nearly every joint by means of these tiny fiberoptic tubes. From the orthopedic surgeon's standpoint, there seemed to be a surgical answer to most chronic musculoskeletal problems. But, as I continued in clinical practice, that wasn't always the case. Nonetheless, the fascination with the engineering and techniques of surgery has kept most orthopedic surgeons focused at surgical solutions. The world of orthopedic medicine is usually essentially ignored.

Orthopedic medicine—the nonsurgical and nonpharmacologic approach to musculoskeletal problems—has had a difficult time in the world of traditional scientific medicine. Evaluation in orthopedic medicine depends of high levels of manual skills that are not easily transferred from the written page or the lecture. Experience and a receptive mental attitude are necessary to develop these evaluation skills. Compounding the difficulty is the fact that beginning and end points of treatments have few objective characteristics. Diminished tenderness, straighter posture, increased energy, and reduced pain complaints are very subjective. In contrast to fractures, each problem is somewhat different as to the location of the weak link. Since anatomy of postural balance, health and stability, and integrated fascial function are all difficult to objectively measure, they were kept from being incorporated into standard orthopedic, physiatric, or even osteopathic training models. From my standpoint as a professor of orthopedic surgery, these concepts were easier to ignore than to incorporate into training. It was easier to say individuals had psychologic barriers than structural barriers that kept them from being well. Because few papers involving concepts related to orthopedic medicine could meet the stringent requirements of the peer reviewed journals, they seldom became visible in the traditional literature. There was little money for research, and the objective measurements needed for a scientific study are very difficult to apply.

Then a funny thing happened. Some of my patients who had failed to benefit from my traditional orthopedic surgical approach received some injections of proliferant solution. These made them better. I thought it must be a hoax or a placebo effect. Nonetheless, since I did not understand the material being injected, I had to investigate it further. To my surprise, a prospective scientific study on prolotherapy was about to be initiated in Santa Barbara, California. I was asked to monitor the study to vouch for the methods and result. I actually took on this role with the confidence that my scientific integrity would be able to squash this "hokey" concept of sclerosant injection into ligaments once and for all. I had heard of it, of course; the same concept had worked for the old-time vascular surgeons. However, none of my professors had ever talked about it, and I had never seen an exhibit at an academy meeting about it. What reason was there to believe it worked? But, I wondered, could it work? Thus, I became involved with a prospective randomized double-blind study in Santa Barbara in otherwise healthy people with chronic back and pelvis pain.[1] This was the best clinical study in which I had ever been involved. To rule out all placebo effect, the results of this prospective study were not evaluated until 6 months after the completion of treatment. The study was described by the editor of the journal *Spine* as an "elegant study." It clearly documented the benefits of prolotherapy over injection of local anesthesia. The editors of *Spine*, however, said they could not publish it, because they did not like the results! Although I was one of the founding editors of *Spine*, I resigned, and the paper was published elsewhere.[1]

This short story underscores the bias in the scientific community against innovative concepts that, by the nature of the tissue being evaluated in treatment, have poor capacity for objective measurement. Good clinical studies are expensive. The small 95-subject Santa Barbara project cost hundreds of thousands of dollars that were provided by a private foundation. A prodigious amount of donated time was necessary to complete it. Can you imagine the government funding a prolotherapy study?

Now, dear reader, it is time for you to judge for yourself. Neat new words will emerge such as *tensegrity, the pelvic gear box, ligamentous, storage and release of energy*, and, particularly, *the integrated fascial system*. The sacroiliac joint will emerge as a major factor in initiating or enhancing chronic low back pain. And, most of all, scientific validity for repair stimulation of ligamentous structures by injections will be offered.

This volume needs to be approached with an open mind. Don't sit down to read it when you are angry with the latest denial by some managed care entity of what you think is appropriate care. Take on this reading with the attitude of looking over the horizon. You won't agree with everything said but will frequently ask yourself: "Why can't that be true?" Many times you will find no argument against the reality of the concepts presented.

I was pleased to respond to Dr. Tom Dorman's request to write an introduction to this valuable volume of innovative and justifiable approaches to the care of the back and pelvis. This approach is safe, works well in appropriate patients, and should be part of the health care system of clinicians interested in comprehensive care of patients. It is also inexpensive. Perhaps, in this era of cost concern, its time has arrived.

REFERENCES

1. Klein RG, Eek BC, DeLong WB, Mooney V: A randomized double-blind trial of dextrose-glycerin-phenol injections for chronic low back pain. J Spinal Disord 6:23–33, 1993.

THOMAS A. DORMAN, MD

OVERVIEW: A NEW UNDERSTANDING OF THE HUMAN PELVIS

Private Practice
San Luis Obispo, California

This chapter summarizes many of the new ideas contained in this volume.

Locomotion and Oscillation

Forward advancement of any organism, in its own medium, be it flight, swimming, or walking, is by a process of cyclic movements. This usually involves more than one organ, whereby energy is restored into the system rhythmically through *oscillation*. The momentum, the flywheel effect, is achieved either through the recoil of elastic tissues or the oscillation of a weight such as a pendulum. The trunk of the bounding cat, the tail of the hopping kangaroo, the limbs of a galloping camel all represent these mechanisms. It was believed until recently that in the case of human walking (in contrast to running) no energy is stored and released.[20] Whether the development of mechanical clocks took its cues from nature is unknown. Regardless, in a pendulum, kinetic and antigravitational potential energy alternate. The clockwork mechanism allows the escapement of the stored (mainspring) energy to be released regularly, rhythmically, and *efficiently* through the use of a pendulum. It was the invention of Christiaan Huygens (1629–1695), a Dutch watchmaker, who was first able to store elastic energy in a spring, liberating reliable time-keeping mechanisms for the first time from what we now call long-case clocks. In the spring-driven escapement we have an analogy to the second *oscillating mechanisms* in locomotion of organisms including that of our own.

Human Walking

Among mammals only *Homo sapiens* is an erect organism.[33] Even apes, the species closest to

SPINE: State of the Art Reviews—Vol. 9, No. 2, May 1995
Philadelphia, Hanley & Belfus, Inc.

313

humans as judged by comparative anatomy, are essentially quadruped creatures, which, like the domestic dog, can rise on their hind legs temporarily. During walking, humans swing their arms. These short pendulums store and release antigravitational energy and contribute to the overall efficiency of the locomotor mechanism, which, in reality, is the whole human body. The arms swing to and aft alternately on the two sides, thereby creating torque through the upper girdle, and in brisk walking the upper girdle rotates alternately with each step versus the pelvis. This torque represents storage and release of elastic energy in the fascial layers of the trunk, particularly the paraspinal ligaments. The lower limbs also serve as pendulums. An easy way to appreciate their role as pendulums is to watch an individual walking on a treadmill. The body is stationary against the surrounding room, and it is easy to see how each leg rises and falls alternately with the other and how the advancement of the trunk of the walking person is not continuous but oscillates depending on the phase in the cycle of movement of the legs. As the swing-leg accelerates, the trunk slows, relatively, and, with planting, that leg decelerates while the trunk speeds up. The trunk accelerates and decelerates with each leg swing cycle. This phenomenon is repeated when the other leg takes over the pendular-swing function. It is evident that the legs have the additional function of stance and that these functions alternate between the sides and within the cycle. How is the energy of momentum, the kinetic energy, transferred from the leg (pendulum) to the trunk? Before answering *how* the forces are transferred, take the example of the *dynamic-passive walker*, a mechano-like assemblage in which the equivalent of a human torso is mounted on "thighs" through a horizontal transverse axle representing "hips." The knees are similarly represented (with extension blocks) and the feet are rockers. This mechanical contraption can imitate human forward walking down a slope angled at 3°, once it is started, without additional energetic input. The kinetic pendular energy of each leg is sufficient, on planting, to transfer sufficient momentum to the torso to lift the second leg off the ground and bring it into swing. This device demonstrates, therefore, that walking is a dynamic-passive attribute of the balance and linkage geometry of the upright human.[19] Taking a stroll on a level surface consumes little effort. Therefore, walking can be achieved through kinetic pendular mechanisms with little energy. The transfer of forces is simply through the mechanical linkages. Clearly, this applies to the human frame, with the pelvis being the relevant *linkage*.

Trying to walk without swinging the trunk or arms is somewhat inconvenient. The swing of the arms and upper trunk is not merely an atavistic neuronal release but a mechanical contribution through an *oscillating mechanism*. At a glance, the efficiency is mechanical, dynamic, and antigravitational. However, elastic energy also must be considered in living organisms. In the dynamic-passive walker, there are no elastic components. On the other hand, the energy stored and released anti-gravitationally by the upper limbs (pendulums) is transferred into a *torque of the trunk*, which, in turn, is applied through ligaments and fasciae that bind the lower lumbar vertebrae and sacrum to the ilia. The torque is transferred diffusely through the soft tissues. The mechanical loci of transfer are the (propeller-shaped) sacroiliac joints. It is through the *sacroiliac mechanism* that the flywheel effect of the rotation of the trunk with its attendant (upper limb) pendulums contributes to the momentum of walking.

The Role of the Pelvis

The construction of this mechanism is predicated on a unique role of the human pelvis. It has the task of combining stability in stance with mobility in swing. The mobility is not merely passive but must allow the release of the stored elastic energy in the fasciae into the other moving parts. It is not surprising, therefore, that the unique joints of the pelvis, the sacroiliac joints, are different anatomically and functionally from all other joints of the body. All other synovial joints are low-friction devices. Although the sacroiliac joint allows a small range of movement, it is a high-friction device analogous to the clutch of a shift-stick automobile. It is in the unique anatomic characteristic that we also find the unique physiologic one: the ability to maintain *force closure* on the stance side and unlock, allowing the transfer of the elastic energy on the swing side.

An understanding of this relationship has developed in the last decade. The recognition of the unique characteristics of the sacroiliac joint, that of force closure, comes from a group in Rotterdam[30,31] (see chapter 10). These researchers tested the friction coefficient of the surfaces of the sacroiliac joint by mechanical means and reviewed the macroscopic and microscopic anatomy of the surfaces. Measurements of the efficiency of walking, by way of assessing oxygen consumption while walking on a treadmill, were performed at California Polytechnic State University in San Luis Obispo, California. Arm swinging, the rise and fall of the trunk, leg swing, and rotation of the trunk were each found to contribute to the efficiency of walking. This was evaluated by measuring the oxygen consumption of each of the individual components and comparing the sum with the actual consumption of oxygen with normal walking.[4]

Sacroiliac Joint Movement

Some erroneous teaching about the sacroiliac joints has occurred in this century. A number of texts have stated that no movement occurs at these joints except in parturition; however, stereophotogrammatic studies[7,16] and radiologic cadaver imaging[32] have demonstrated movement at these joints. In life, movement has been demonstrated by placing Kirschner nails in the sacrum and ilium and watching the movement in walking individuals.[2] The range of movement and the axis of rotation, however, are extraordinarily variable among individuals, a finding that is not surprising considering the extraordinary variability in the anatomy of the joints themselves.[28] This is an example where a reductionist analysis of movement, the analogy with moving mechanical devices, fails. The forces are transmitted through the soft tissues, and attempts to analyze the mechanics in a manner analogous to that of moving parts and machinery have been unproductive. The *instantaneous access of rotation* is a term used by engineers to define the mechanical relationship between irregularly moving surfaces predicated on the tension of the soft tissues. This writer has found this approach not useful from a biologic and medical perspective.

Pelvic Dysfunction

A person standing on one leg does not fall down. The vertical poise against gravity is predicated on balance: the upper part of the body is broader than the base (foot). The ability to maintain balance in one-legged stance is an achievement that physicists call *unstable equilibrium*; minor sways of the body are countered by muscle action that brings the center of gravity back over the narrow base. The brain senses the balance and commands the muscles. The second factor that allows balance is the stability of the leg. One would think that the stable strut would best be made of a pillar of bone. However, the foot is actually mounted through the hinge of the ankle by the tibia, and the femur is mounted on top of it through another hinge. The ball and socket of the hip is superseded by the last joint in this chain, the sacroiliac joint. The (floppy) spine is mounted on top. How is it, then, that this loose jointed collection of bones serves as a pillar? The joints facilitate locomotion, and there is a need for stability and mobility in the same structure.

Although this chapter concentrates on pelvic dysfunction, a brief review of the other section of the pillar is presented. The foot is planted and the leg hinges over the ankle as a person walks over the stance foot. During this phase the knee is locked in (hyper) extension, which converts the hinge to a solid leg as long as the force of gravity maintains the slight hyperextending pressure. The quadriceps muscle guards this position, but in a normal knee stability is maintained passively by the ligaments. In the case of the ball and socket of the hip joint, as long as the femur is upright, the acetabulum has nowhere to go. When standing on one leg, whether you allow your pelvis to sag (in the Trendelenburg position) or whether you hoist your body over your standing femur, the righting reflex maintains the center of gravity right over the leg, so that only slight muscular action is needed.

Stability at the sacroiliac joint is based on a more complex mechanism, which has recently been called *self-bracing*[27] (see chapter 10). This is an excellent term but is conceptually little different from the *ex-center* stability maintained through the knee. The sacroiliac joint is a synovial joint that, in contrast to the other synovial joints of the body, has a rough surface. This has been demonstrated both microscopically and macroscopically.[19] When the auricular surface is inspected frontally it has, as the name indicates, the approximate appearance of a pinna. It appears L-shaped, open backward. The major stabilizing ligament of this joint, which is the thickest ligament in the human frame, is located at the elbow of the L. The collagenous fibers of this ligament are intertwined diagonally as they traverse the short distance between the bones. The surfaces of the sacroiliac joints are not oriented in any of the primary body planes. The ilial surface faces medially, forward, and superiorly. The joint is not planar in adults. The medial, superior, and anterior facing applies to the upper (and larger) section of the joint. The inferior part is even more variable than the superior, but modally usually faces medially, posteriorly, and superiorly. The joint surface is similar to a propeller or a corkscrew; the geometry of screws is best defined by the direction in which they tighten. Tightening between the sacrum and ilium in the case of the sacroiliac joint is not dissimilar. In contrast to a wood screw, the tightening of the sacroiliac joint is controlled by the main central ligament (which can be thought of as a rope). As torque is applied, the fibers are squeezed together and the rope tightens. Because the rope is short, the ilium and sacrum are forced together. The rough surfaces between them maintain stable approximation; hence the stability when weight is borne on one leg.

The direction of closure and tightening of the surfaces of the sacroiliac joint is based on its geometry. Closure is achieved as the superior end of the sacrum moves backward against the ilium. This has been defined as *counternutation*. It is instinctual to think of rotation as around an axis, but the movement of most joints consists of a combination of rotation and gliding.[24] To maintain their terminology of rotation, engineers have coined the term *instantaneous axis of rotation* to define the minute fraction of the movement that has a theoretical axis at each degree of movement. This "point" moves with the glide, so they speak of a *moving instantaneous axis of rotation*. The interrelationship of these axes are a physicist's Ptolemaic calculus. To the clinician the action is in the ligaments. Tightening through a twist is achieved here, and the bony surfaces are approximated. There is an extraordinary degree of variation in the detailed bony anatomy between individuals and even between the two sides. In any case the geometry of the joint goes through changes with aging.

The function remains the same during the walking phase of life. So in walking, through counternutation, with approximation of the bones and a variable glide of the auricular surfaces on each other, stability of the pillar is maintained during the stance phase. The pillar reverts to a flexible pendulum as the stride advances and the leg alternates into the swing phase; the knee unlocks, flexion occurs at the hip, and at the sacroiliac joint nutation occurs on that side; the sacroiliac ligament unwinds a little (incidentally restoring some elastic energy into the mechanism of locomotion) as the ilium moves slightly backward and medially on the sacrum.

The mechanism of locking at the sacroiliac joints alternates between the sides, locking on the stance side and unlocking on the swing side. Efficient walking is predicated on the mechanism being reliable. The fidelity consists of maintaining a stable strut in stance and unlocking on cue.

In the case of the movement of the peripheral joints, locking in stability, where it occurs, is dependent on position and the forces surrounding the joint but not dependent directly on the function of another joint. The sacroiliac joints are not so lucky, because they share the sacrum. Even this versatile bone can move only in one direction at a time. Additionally, the ilia are united anteriorly at the syndesmosis of the symphysis. Herein lies the weakness of the human pelvis. In normal walking the sacroiliac joints lock and unlock on either side alternately so that counternutation (locking) and nutation (unlocking) define the cyclic sequence. The phases are opposite on the two sides. Since locking consists of a backward movement of the upper portion of the sacrum[10] versus the ilium, if locking were to occur simultaneously on both sides, there would be extreme counternutation of the sacrum versus both ilia. Because of the angle of the sacroiliac joint in the coronal plane, the pelvic circumference would tend to enlarge. The ligaments will allow so much stretch that as the sacrum gets wedged backward between the two ilia, the ligaments are finally tightened. Due to the locking mechanism discussed earlier, it is possible for the sacrum to become *trapped* in this position. The inferior surfaces of the sacroiliac joints are such that for entrapment at the lower level of the pelvis to occur (as seen in the coronal plane) the inferior surface of the sacrum would need to move forward between the two ilia (this is also defined in the movement of counternutation). Since there is no distinct axis of rotation, the phenomenon of self-bracing, with entrapment of both sacroiliac joints (through counternutation of the sacrum bilaterally), can occur in the upper portion of the pelvic ring, the level of the inferior portion of the sacroiliac joints, or at both simultaneously.

To complicate matters, entrapment can occur when the ilia are aligned symmetrically about each other or when one is relatively more forward than the other. The usual situation is an anterior right ilium in right-handed individuals.[15] Ligaments are elastic. When stretched, the abducting forces contained in the elasticity of the ligaments of the pelvic ring, particularly the posterior sacroiliac ligaments, tend to maintain the entrapment. The self-bracing mechanism of the sacroiliac joint, through its propeller shape and rough surfaces, partakes in this entrapment. Therefore, when both legs are in the stance phase of locomotion simultaneously, this phenomenon of pelvic entrapment can occur. Conceptually this is no more complicated than driving a wedge into a tight space. Attempts to define the various possible positions of the three pelvic bones in relation to each other have proved difficult over the past century, and the relationships have been systematized only recently.[11] Anterior rotation of the ilia, on one or both sides relative to the sacrum, is believed to be common in persons with back pain and is the cause of most pelvic dysfunction. This dysfunction is responsible for many remote secondary soft tissue strains often defined as local areas of *somatic dysfunction*. Manual correction, followed by self treatments of the anterior rotation and strengthening of the abdominal muscles, relieves the problem in most patients.[3] The first clinical observation usually is the loss of lordosis with pain in attempted extension at the lumbosacral level while standing. The usual range (for that patient) of rotation and side bending is also reduced, because the slack, usually present in the ligaments, which would ordinarily allow these movements, is taken up by the abnormal (entrapped) position of the sacrum.[29] The importance of the slack in the soft tissues was described first in the case of cross-referred pain from dysfunction in the sacroiliac joints in pain from attempted straight leg raising.[21] Pseudo-leg-length-discrepancy on lying supine is usual, but it also can be found in individuals without pain. The presence of the asymmetry in normal persons, while it becomes more pronounced in patients with entrapment, has been called *asymlocation*.[6]

In the frontal plane the sacrum is seen as wider at its cephalic end. This has led to the time-honored impression that it functions like a *keystone* in an arch. Although this observation seems to be correct only when it is in *dysfunction*, this practitioner has observed that patients with pelvic dysfunction lose up to 2 cm in height when their pelvis is dysfunctional. Some height is regained after successful manipulation. This observation supports the notion that the sacrum descends between the ilia with wedging and, at least in some instances, with entrapment.

The human pelvis in mechanically unique. The phenomenon of entrapment through the maintained adducting forces of the elastic ligaments, which hold the three pelvic bones together, can last for long times. When the sacrum is firmly entrapped this way, the patient becomes dependent on an *external force*—manipulation—to unlock the dysfunction. When the degree of entrapment is less severe, maneuvers that patients can do themselves might suffice to restore optimal symmetry or at least reduce the severity of the dysfunction. This phenomenon of entrapment, of *somatic dysfunction*, is characteristic of but not confined to the human pelvis. Pelvic dysfunction is, however, usually present when somatic dysfunction exists at any level of the axial skeleton. It is persistent or recurrent unless the pelvis is restored to normal. This author suggests that the reason is the *unique quality of the human pelvis— entrapment*. The aphorism that *pain is a liar* can be attributed to the fact that through the transfer of the tension in ligaments and fascia, the strain might be felt at a distant site.

Bipedality, by its inherent nature, necessitates alternating stance and swing phases of the legs. The transfer of weight from the central axial skeleton alternately to the legs is responsible for the inexorable mechanics of the human pelvis. These mechanics are quite different from those of all other creatures. The other bipedal animals, birds and, once, dinosaurs, have different mechanics because they balance their tail and trunk like a see-saw; in contrast, humans balance the vertical torso over a point.

Therefore, a mechanical analysis of the function of ligaments affords an understanding of the dynamic forces active in locomotion and explains both the function and dysfunction of the *unique* human pelvis. This author proposes that future medical texts should contain a section on ligaments with a subsection on disordered mechanics after a suitable analysis of normal mechanics. The chapter headings regarding the management of dysfunction should include manipulation because only manipulation can release entrapment. The altered strength and elasticity of ligaments should be addressed. The available modalities of treatment include (1) an adjustment in frequency of usage (rest and exercise), (2) metabolic support systemically (nutrition), (3) and local approaches (prolotherapy[25]). Preventive measures should include advice about maintaining satisfactory alignment of mechanics. Perhaps ligament weakness can be attributed to a sedentary lifestyle punctuated with acceleration deceleration forces on the axial skeleton. Does posture play a role? There seems to be less back pain in primitive societies. It has been suggested that forces transferred via the hamstrings and the sacrotuberous ligament to the inferolateral angle of the sacrum, tending to bring on nutation, are present during squatting while maintaining lordosis of the lumbar spine.[18] These forces might serve pelvic alignment and training better than sitting in a chair. Is it possible that the epidemic of back pain in western civilization is a side effect of comfortable furniture and the toilet seat?

Prolotherapy and Manipulation

Hyperplasia of collagenous tissue can be achieved through stimulating inflammation. Indeed, the process of inflammation originally defined by Eli Metchnikoff[23] and subsequently studied by Cohnheim[1] is known as the source of organismal repair. Every surgeon relies on this inflammation for wound repair in anticipation of suture removal. It has been known since the days of Hippocrates[13] that the irritation of fibrous tissue can provoke hypertrophy. (The following chapter describes the history of wound repair from Hippocrates to the present day.)

The role of manual therapy has been subject to controversial argumentation to a large extent because of the mindset of establishment medicine that was introduced with the reorganization of medicine in 1910.[8] Its usefulness has gained recognition through the force of the marketplace and was reported to constitute, in chiropractic hands alone, a $4.5 billion dollar yearly industry in 1991.[17] Only recently has scientific writing yielded a small place in the de jure scientific pantheon to what is de facto a common experience of most individuals who have suffered back pain and have been treated manually.[26]

Combined Management of Back Pain

Despite the possible limitations of the reductionist approach, the use of diagnosis has remained central in orthopedic medicine. The cardinal characteristics of ligaments are clinical manifestations of dysfunction, which have been defined elsewhere.[6] In summary, persistent pain from maintenance of tension for long periods *(posain)* and a false sensation of a numb-like feeling *(nulliness)* have been recognized (see chapter 3). These terms have been used in the last half decade seemingly propitiously. It should be noted that ligaments lend themselves to imaging poorly, dysfunction does not have an imaging counterpart at all in these structures, and there are no laboratory tests for abnormal ligaments. Therefore, clinicians must rely on their bedside skills and a knowledge of anatomy, both of which are waning in an age of the quick fix, the reductionist approach, and molecular biology.

Ongley's Technique

The combination of manipulation with ligament refurbishing, or prolotherapy, can be seen as the logical outcome of this discussion. We owe, however, to the genius of Ongley the combination of manipulation with prolotherapy and a number of additional essential components creating what is called the *Ongley technique*. This approach is appropriate only in cases in which the diagnosis of persistent somatic dysfunction in the pelvis is confirmed and in which more significant disease has been excluded. Does the refurbishment of the posterior sacroiliac ligaments with prolotherapy work? The clinical effectiveness has been subject to two clinical trials,[14,25] and the mechanical changes in the alignment of the iliac bones versus each other, tending to symmetry with treatment, also has been shown. It also has been found that the efficiency of walking, as judged by oxygen consumption, improves after treatment.[5] This observation ties the treatment by Ongley's technique into the new understanding of the role of the pelvis in locomotion.

The Slipping Clutch Syndrome

A number of individuals in back pain clinics report episodic falling. The leg gives way when entering into stance irregularly and unexpectedly. This is an *intrinsic injury*.[22] The patient's reaction is one of embarrassment, and persistent dysfunction is never seen. The clinician must separate these episodes of falling from other causes of loss of function such as epilepsy, cardiac arrhythmia, and loose bodies and joints. These episodes of falling have cleared up in a number patients treated with prolotherapy to the posterior sacroiliac joint ligaments. Therefore, it was realized through serendipity that the falling (dysfunction) was due to momentary slippage of the sacroiliac joint (clutch) as individuals entered into stance, which caused them to lose balance and fall. No defect of the central nervous system can be detected in these cases. The sobriquet given to this condition, the *slipping clutch syndrome*, is an attempt at an analysis of the cause as well as a shorthand description.

Summary

The tenets of this chapter are as follows:

1. The human pelvis is unique in bipedal locomotion. Its function is that of a gearbox transferring forces for the enhanced efficiency of walking.

2. The efficiency of walking is predicated on the flywheel effect of the moving parts.

3. Antigravitational pendular limb movements contribute to the storage and release of energy.

4. Elastic recoil in ligaments and fasciae throughout the body contribute to the storage and release of energy.

5. The ligamentous fascial organ functions as a whole.

6. Dysfunction of the clockwork, or transducer-like role of the pelvis, is predicated on its unique delicate balance.

7. With persistent dysfunction, in addition to pain, there is inefficiency in walking.

8. Dysfunction at the sacroiliac joint can manifest itself by mechanical failure, the slipping clutch syndrome, and with pain.

9. An understanding of the mechanics and mechanical dysfunction explains the effectiveness of the two clinical tools.

10. The clinical tools for dealing with the problems (in addition to correct diagnosis) are manipulation and prolotherapy.

11. *Tensegrity* is the term used to convey the phenomenon of transferred forces through a structure constituted of tension and compression members, like the skeletal ligamentous system. Therefore, an understanding of tensegrity is required in management.

REFERENCES

1. Cohnheim JF: Lectures on General Pathology (English translation). New York, Dover Publications, 1968 (original, London, 1889).
2. Colachis SC, Worden RE, Bechtol CO, et al: Movement of the sacro-iliac joint in the adult male: A preliminary report. Arch Phys Med Rehabil 44:1963.

3. DonTigny RL: Sacroiliac dysfunction: Recognition and treatment. First Interdisciplinary World Congress on Low Back Pain and its Relation to the Sacroiliac Joint. San Diego, November 5–6, 1992. Rotterdam, ECO, 1992, pp 481–517.

4. Dorman TA, Buchmiller JC, Cohen RE, et al: Energy efficiency during human walking. J Orthop Med 15:64–67, 1993.

5. Dorman TA, Cohen RE, Dasig D, et al: Energy efficiency during human walking; before and after prolotherapy. J Orthop Med 17:24–26, 1995.

6. Dorman TA, Ravin T: Diagnosis and Injection Techniques in Orthopedic Medicine. Baltimore, Williams & Wilkins, 1991.

7. Egund N, Olsson TH, Schmid H, et al: Movement in the sacro-iliac joints demonstrated with Roentgen stereophotogrammetry. Acta Radiol Diagn 19:833–845, 1978.

8. Flexner A: Medical Education in the United States and Canada. A report to the Carnegie Foundation for the Advancement of Teaching, 1910. The Carnegie Foundation, 1910.

9. Gedney EH: Hypermobile joint. Osteopathic Profession 4:30–31, 1937.

10. Greenman PE: Clinical aspects of sacroiliac function in walking. J Man Med 5:125–130, 1990.

11. Greenman PE: Principles of Manual Medicine. Baltimore, Williams & Wilkins, 1989.

12. Hackett GS: Ligament and Tendon Relaxation treated By Prolotherapy. 3rd ed. Springfield, IL, Charles C. Thomas, 1958.

13. Hippocrates: The Genuine Works of Hippocrates (Francis Adams, trans.). Baltimore, Williams & Wilkins, 1946.

14. Klein RG, Eek BJ, DeLong B, Mooney V: A randomized double-blind trial of dextrose-glycerine-phenol injections for chronic low back pain. J Spinal Disord 6:22–23, 1993.

15. LaCourse M, Moore K, Davis K, et al: A report on the asymmetry of iliac inclination: A study comparing normal, laterality and change in a patient population with painful sacro-iliac dysfunction treated with prolotherapy. J Orthop Med 12:69–72, 1990.

16. Lavignolle B, Vital JM, Senegas J, et al: An approach to the functional anatomy of the sacroiliac joints in vivo. Anat Clin 5:169–176, 1983.

17. Lawrence DJ: Chiropractic Diagnosis and Management. Baltimore, Williams & Wilkins, 1991.

18. Martin RM: The Gravity Guiding System. San Marino, CA, Essential Publishing, 1975.

19. McGeer T: Passive dynamic walking. Int J Robotics Res 9:62–82, 1990.

20. McNeil AR: Elastic Mechanism in Animal Movement. New York, Cambridge University Press, 1988.

21. Mennell J: Back Pain. Boston, Little, Brown & Co.,1960.

22. Mennell JM. Joint Pain. Boston, Little, Brown & Co., 1964.

23. Metchnikoff E: Lectures on the Comparative Pathology of Inflammation. New York, Dover Publications, 1968 (original, 1893).

24. Miller JAA, Schultz AB, Andersson GBJ: Load-displacement behavior of sacroiliac joints. J Orthop Res 5:92–101, 1987.

25. Ongley MJ, Klein RG, Dorman TA, et al. A new approach to the treatment of chronic back pain. Lancet 2:143–146, 1987.

26. Shekelle, PG, Adams, AH, Chassin, MR, et al: Spinal manipulation for low-back pain. Ann Intern Med 117:590–598, 1992.

27. Snijders CJ, Vleeming A, Stoeckart R: Transfer of lumbosacral load to iliac bones and legs. Part 1. Biomechanics of self-bracing of the sacroiliac joints and its significance for treatment and exercise. First Interdisciplinary World Congress on Low Back Pain and its Relation to the Sacroiliac Joint. San Diego, November 5–6, 1992. Rotterdam, ECO, 1992, pp 233–254.

28. Solonen KA: The sacroiliac joint in the light of anatomical, roentgenological and clinical studies. Acta Orthop Scand Suppl 1957.

29. Stevens A: Side bending in axial rotation of the sacrum inside the pelvic girdle. First Interdisciplinary World Congress on Low Back Pain and its Relation to the Sacroiliac Joint. San Diego, November 5–6, 1992. Rotterdam, ECO, 1992, pp 209–230.

30. Vleeming A, Stoeckart R, Volkers AC, Snijders CJ: Relation between form and function in the sacroiliac joint. Part I: Clinical anatomical aspects. Spine 15:130–132, 1990.

31. Vleeming, Volkers AC, Snijders CJ, Stoeckart R: Relation between form and function in the sacroiliac joint. Part II: Biomechanical aspects. Spine 15:133–136, 1990.

32. Weisl H. The movement of the sacro-iliac joint. Acta Anat 23:80–91, 1955.

33. Wolff HD: Comments on the evolution of the sacroiliac joint in progress and vertebral column research. First International Symposium on the Sacroiliac Joint, Its Role in Posture and Locomotion. Rotterdam, ECO, 1991.

THOMAS A. DORMAN, MD

CONCEPTS IN ORTHOPEDIC MEDICINE

Private Practice
San Luis Obispo, California

Portions of this chapter have been excerpted from Dorman TA: Storage and release of elastic energy in the pelvis: Dysfunction, diagnosis, and treatment. J Orthop Med 14:54–62, 1992; with permission.

The discussion of concepts represents a challenge and an opportunity. This volume introduces new concepts and attempts to kindle an understanding of orthopedic medicine and, in particular, the injection technique called *prolotherapy* in the "thought tools" of busy, efficient practitioners. Orthopedic medicine is a branch of medicine first defined by James Cyriax in 1929 and developed through the eight editions of his textbook.[4] The need for this branch was not appreciated in America when medicine was modernized and organized into its current format[8] in 1910 by Abraham Flexner on behalf of the Carnegie Foundation. The incidence of ligamentous and fascial injuries seems to be increasing.[5] Since this issue focuses on spinal conditions, the reader is referred to the original texts[3] of Cyriax regarding peripheral joints. Additional concepts have grown with the profession and are discussed in subsequent sections of this chapter.

The thought tools doctors use and refer to as *concepts* are reviewed below. From Ayn Rand, we learn:

According to objectivism, concepts "represent classifications of observed existents according to their relationships to other observed existents." To form a concept one mentally *isolates* a group of concretes (of distinct perceptual units), on the basis of observed similarities which distinguish them from all other known concretes (similarities is "the relationship between two or more existents which possess the same characteristic(s), but in different measure or degree"); by a process of omitting the particular measurements of these concretes, one integrates them into a single new mental unit: the concept, which subsumes all

SPINE: State of the Art Reviews—Vol. 9, No. 2, May 1995
Philadelphia, Hanley & Belfus, Inc.

323

concretes of this kind (a potentially unlimited number). The integration is completed and retained by the selection of a perceptual symbol (a word) to designate it. "A concept is a mental integration of two or more units possessing the same distinguishing characteristic(s), with their particular measurements omitted."[19]

In what context should the new concepts suggested here be viewed? Orthopedic medicine lies full square in the tradition of rationalist, or allopathic, medicine. But like other sections of allopathic medicine, it has borrowed from the empiricist tradition.[2] These borrowings constitute a psychological barrier in certain circles. The rationalist tradition traces its origins to Greek medicine. Since then, we have discarded many of the specifics, such as phlebotomy, and concepts, such as humors. However, Greek medicine remains the basis of our thought tools. Praxagoras (about 350 BC) was the first to define entities that vary from health. From him comes the quintessence of the concepts of disease and diagnosis.[21] Paracelsus (1493–1541) can be credited with our understanding of the origins of the concepts of our rationalist, experimental, scientific, contemporary method. Paracelsus realized that the laws of nature are observations and used the term *practica globulae* for them. While he recognized the limitations of experiments in the absence of an hypothesis, he was the first to appreciate the deficiency of unconfirmed ideas and theories—scholastic speculation. Modern science is based on experimentation, which, in turn, is based on the evolution of hypothesis.[21] We owe to Paracelsus the distillation of a rationalist thread in civilization at a time when the minds of men were awash with superstitions, the effluvium of the Dark Ages. An early landmark is anatomic research in the vivisection of condemned criminals, which occurred in Alexandria.[7] Erasistratos was also credited with performing the first physiologic experiment. He placed a bird in a glass jar without feeding it. Upon removal, the bird and its excrements were found to weigh less than the bird alone at the outset of the experiment. It is on the basis of this tradition, the combination of clinical observations, the development of hypothesis, the design of an anatomic or physiologic experiment, and, finally, the testing of hypothesis, that knowledge advances. The contemporary definition of the empiric method[20] stylized this rationale. In this book, the reader can trace these same elements, reflecting the advancement of knowledge in orthopedic medicine. Orthopedic medicine is still in the formative phase, a phase through which other branches of medicine have already passed.

Rationalist physicians are apt to perceive the disease and not the patient. Holistic physicians (and, as an extreme example, homeopaths) treat the constitutional characteristics of the subject, hoping that symptoms will dissipate therefrom. Osteopaths rearrange axial alignment, optimally hoping that remote symptoms in the musculoskeletal system (and elsewhere) will dissipate. Where in this matrix do orthopedic physicians fit? They fit in the rationalist tradition, using concepts from holism and osteopathy. The dysfunctions, or diseases, recognized in orthopedic medicine are singular with unique manifestations. They fall into distinct patterns that have emerged from *syndrome* into *disease* and to which the conceptual tools of *treatment, indications, therapeutic ratio*, and others apply.

Restriction in Movement

John Mennell classified the barriers of joint movements[16] defining voluntary (physiologic) and passive (anatomic) ranges. He also recognized joint play, involuntary movements in joints that differ from their prime motion. Restrictions or barriers can affect a joint diffusely (nonspecifically), and this has been defined by James

Cyriax[3] as the *capsular pattern*. In contrast, restrictions that differ from those caused by a general shrinkage of joint capsules are "nonanatomic" and have been defined as *noncapsular*. In parallel, and seemingly unrelated, the concept of the *osteopathic lesion*, later redefined as *somatic dysfunction*,[11] has arisen in reference to the spine. As pointed out in chapter 13, it might be possible to merge the terminology from these disparate sources in orthopedic medicine because the *concept* is the same. What is the cause of the asymmetric functional barrier in the axial skeleto-ligamentous-fascial organ we call the spine? There is probably more than one cause. However, the unifying factor is almost certainly in the soft tissues, the ligaments, and fasciae. The mechanism of the transfer of forces within these structures, the *tensegrity mechanism*, is altered asymmetrical tension (see chapters 5 and 7). The human pelvis might be thought of as a mechanical trap because of the unique nature of the sacroiliac articulations. It is therefore not surprising that it is a common osteopathic experience that whenever somatic dysfunction is identified anywhere in the body, and certainly in the trunk, pelvic dysfunction is present. As discussed in the chapter on self-locking of the sacroiliac articulation (chapter 9), the *transduction* (transfer of forces through the unique function of the human pelvis) is the ultimate (teleological) reason for this phenomenon. An understanding of these concepts is the essence of this review.

Asymlocation

A universal link in machinery is a unit that transmits forces or torque while allowing free movement in several directions through a series of couplings. The body has the same requirement. Connections exist in the body that approximate these models, and they consist of two or more joints usually around one "universal link" bone. There are only a few instances in human anatomy where an intervening bone has *no* muscular or tendinous attachments at all—for example, the lunate or talus. However, there are a few instances in the axial skeleton where one of the bones is almost free of tendon and muscle attachments and is prone to what the author has termed *asymlocation*, like a universal link (Fig. 1). The best examples are the atlas

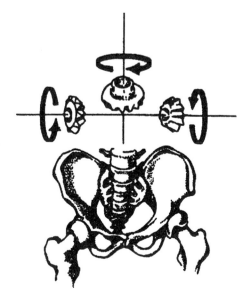

FIGURE 1. Asymlocation of the pelvic area.

and the sacrum, although the lower lumbar vertebrae (usually the fifth) are also prone to this phenomenon. When asymmetric tensions of the surrounding retaining part—for instance, the lumbodorsal fascia—is present, the universal links are apt to be situated with a degree of asymmetry that exceeds the usual or normal and can be a source of dysfunction and pain.

It seems obvious that the sacrum is suspended from the ilia in the quadruped position. This can be appreciated by viewing the pelvic skeleton of any quadruped mammal or viewing the arrangement in the human model in the quadruped position. What is the function of the sacrum in biped standing? The word *function* is used here broadly to discuss the forces controlling it. The sacrum has been compared to the keystone of an architectural arch, which is a uniquely stable arrangement. The vertical forces enhance the stability of the masonry. The greater the weight on the arch, the more stable it is. This is because the adherence of the high friction surfaces between the stones cut into trapezoid forms is enhanced. Does the sacrum indeed function as a keystone in any circumstance at all?

It is a commonplace observation that humans are a little asymmetric. Not only are the internal organs distributed this way, but some asymmetry seems to be more common than not (normal in allopathic terminology in the sense that it is usual) in what has been loosely termed the *soma*. A recent survey of the inclination of the pelvis in healthy athletes has demonstrated that the right ilium is rotated forward in osteopathic terminology normally in right-handed individuals versus the left in left-footed ones. Anyone taking a class in osteopathic manipulation will have observed seemingly healthy class members who have multiple asymmetries in the pelvis and spine, which are described as *somatic dysfunction*. In this sense, *dysfunction* describes what is usual or normal. Another common observation in osteopathic and chiropractic circles is that when these asymmetries are abolished by manual methods in symptomatic individuals, the "dysfunction" is often corrected. In this context, dysfunction and disease bear a proximity. What about the "dysfunction" in asymptomatic individuals? The term *asymlocation* has been proposed by this author[6] for this situation. It seems best suited to describe this circumstance, and it is proposed here that when asymlocation is marked, the propensity to pain (dysfunction) is increased. In contrast, as the dysfunction of the retaining structures (ligaments and fasciae) is healed, asymlocation diminishes. This framework may help to bridge the gap between osteopathy and allopathic medicine.

The Sacroiliac Joints as Friction Absorbers

The irregularities of the auricular surfaces were recognized by early anatomists and the relation to age defined precisely,[15] but only recently have the qualities of the two opposing cartilaginous surfaces of this joint been demonstrated to function as friction devices. This has been demonstrated in gross anatomy and microscopically. The surfaces of the sacroiliac joints function differently from that of other synovial joints. They absorb movement by gliding with friction. They encourage stability rather than free movement[24] (see chapter 10). Therefore, when forces are acting across these joints in a direction other than pure shear, they are apt to offer a high resistance.

Self-Bracing

The forces acting in the pelvis in the upright biped position are self-bracing. The keystone of the arch, the sacrum, being wider superiorly, trends downward from the weight of the body. The traction this applies to the ilia—through the posterior sacroiliac ligaments—tends to bring the ilia into adduction. The wedge shape of the sacrum overall, being wider in front, tends to displace it anteriorly (into the pelvis). A balance occurs between the forward vector and the downward vector. Regardless of the balance, the adducting forces are enhanced through both of these vectors. Because of the bracing mechanism and the posterior sacroiliac ligaments, the sacrum does not descend into the standing pelvis. Self-bracing, therefore, is a unique characteristic of the biped human pelvis.

Self-bracing also applies while standing on both legs. However, since walking predominantly consists of one leg support alternating continuously, self-bracing is switched on and off in gait. Each sacroiliac joint is locked and unlocked with each step alternately, and the joint on the stance side is braced. These presumptions await further confirmation from the laboratory, but the recent demonstration of the production of torque at the sacroiliac articulations with one-legged weightbearing[22] can also be taken to imply the reverse, i.e., the dissipation of the stored (torque) energy into the swing leg with step off. It is proposed here that there is a regular transmission of energy back and forth with locomotion, contributing to the efficiency of the "walking machine."

A clinician listening to the histories of patients with painful backs frequently hears an account that seems to fall into place or match the picture drawn so far. (Perhaps this is the intuitive first step in forming a hypothesis; subsequent experiments may confirm or deny it.) The typical story many sufferers of back pain recount is that their problem began with a major injury. The pain is eventually relieved, sometimes with the help of manipulation. The pain is usually in the low back in the midline, often with radiation into one buttock and possibly down the posterior aspect of the lower limb on the same side. The radiation sometimes alternates between the sides. After a period of normality, lesser and even trivial injuries are apt to reprovoke the pain, which usually recurs in cycles. When taking a detailed history of the provoking event, it is usual to hear that the pain started as the patient was arising from the stooped position and often in an unguarded moment. The onset of pain is unexpected. What is taking place? It is proposed here that the self-bracing or the adducting forces of the ilia come into play as the sacrum moves from the "function" of being suspended to that of being entrapped as a keystone, and, if in the presence of some ligamentous laxity, the transition is not in optimal symmetry, self-bracing occurs before the sacrum can adopt the symmetrical position in the vertical stand. Once self-bracing occurs, muscle spasm aggravates and maintains it. It is the muscle spasm that usually attracts the clinician's attention, but the muscle spasm usually is secondary to the *intrinsic injury* (a term coined by John Mennell[16]).

The Use of Hypothesis

Assuming that asymlocation and self-bracing are commonly the cause of dysfunction and chronic back pain (recurrent and later becoming continuous) and that objective confirmation from the laboratory is not forthcoming, what can the clinician do? From the above discussion, the question is rhetorical: (1) the clinician should restore correct alignment of the axial skeleton, in this case correct the somatic dysfunction of the sacrum between the ilia; (2) take whatever action is necessary to maintain the correction. Hence the idea that appropriate manipulation to restore symmetry to the pelvis might be followed by ligament refurbishment: prolotherapy. This working hypothesis served as the model for the now well-known clinical trial of Ongley's technique.[18] Ongley is owed not only an understanding of the mechanisms discussed above but also the development of the combined technique for treatment. However, the simple application of one type of treatment to all patients with back pain, although it will be effective in many, is neither rational nor wise. Not all back pain has one cause. Therefore, meticulous diagnosis is essential in orthopedic medicine.

Points of Weakness

The concentration of strain always occurs at the weak point, as is seen in a frayed halyard or in the wear and tear of clothing. The weak point itself is always where the rope was damaged first. Clinicians have observed the same phenomenon in the inner lining, the fascia: the strains in the moving parts of the body tend to concentrate and eventually lead to injuries at internal sites, which have patterns. The patterns have mechanical origins that may or may not be able to be analyzed mathematically, intellectually, or intuitively. Nonetheless, the patterns are recognizable to clinicians.

Tensegrity

The form of the body is maintained, in part, by *tensegrity*, a phenomenon that can be appreciated by contemplating a geodesic dome.[9] Variation in the tension of one component of the system affects the whole. This principle is retained in the tensegrity model, and these properties of tensegrity models will become of great importance in research of the fascioligamentous mechanical body system. Although not all mechanical characteristics of the body can be understood through this analogy, it serves to explain many of the observations that have been mysterious. Why, for instance, do so many individuals with whiplash to the neck develop low back pain and vice versa? If the spine is seen as a tensegrity model (picture a garden hose twisted at one end), one can intuitively appreciate that torque will be transmitted to the other end and that straightening the first end will not necessarily straighten the second once the kink has been established in the fabric.

In summary, it is proposed that the pelvic girdle serves as a transmission and differential in locomotion, that the initiating energy arises in muscles, and transmission is through fasciae and ligaments. The transfer of energy from glycogen to distance in walking is modulated by an escapement analogous to that of a clock. A major component of the efficient mechanism is in the elastic storage of energy in ligaments and fasciae proportionate to their abundance. A reductionist quantification of the tension in each fiber relevant to each phase of walking awaits further research.

DIAGNOSIS

The anatomic diagnosis of somatic dysfunction and manual methods of correction are covered best in osteopathic texts and instructional courses.[1,11] What of the direct effects of ligament and fascial strains? A few clinical tools should be used. The following comments refer to some new terms, which are covered extensively elsewhere.[6]

Referred Pain, Posain, and Nulliness

Clinical observations show that mesenchymal structures have characteristic patterns of referred pain, that strained structures may have more than one pattern, and that these patterns do not match injuries in spinal roots, plexuses, trunks, or nerve distributions (Figs. 2 and 3). Whether the patterns are due to errors of perception in the cerebral cortex or have some other atavistic or mechanistic origin is unknown. This ignorance, however, does not alter clinical experience.

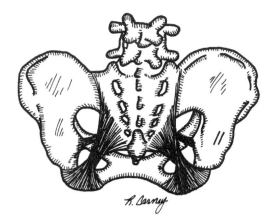

FIGURE 2.   Sacrotuberous ligaments.

A characteristic of strained ligaments maintained under strain is that prolonged stretch provokes the pain of the characteristic distribution alluded to above. Patients will report they are unable to maintain one position for a long time. The term *posain* has been used for this clinical observation.

Another observation is that patients will report numbness in a certain part of the body. The distribution of this symptom is similar to that of posain and when objective testing is undertaken, such as two-point discrimination or nerve conduction studies, no deficit is found. Patients will report that stroking the affected area is either neutral or comfortable. Experientially this observation is so germane that dismissing these patient complaints as aberrations is not tenable. The term *nulliness* describes this phenomenon.

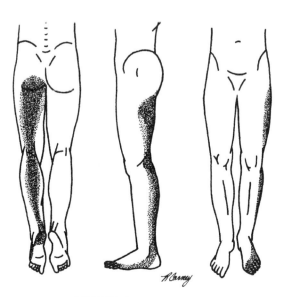

FIGURE 3.   The pain pattern.

TREATMENT

With this conceptual model in mind (many of the ideas are still experimental) a treatment plan falls into place. Sites of ligament or fascial pain need to be identified. The tools for such identification arise on the one hand from an allopathic approach—the analysis of symptoms and a recognition of patterns of referred pain—and on the other from a framework analysis—the tools the osteopath uses in a structural analysis harking back to the teaching of Andrew Still.[23] Using a combination of the skills from both of these professions, an orthopedic physician can advance the clinical diagnosis best.

A tenet of orthopedic medicine is that diagnosis comes first, and the tools of treatment are the restoration of symmetry to the extent that it is possible by methods such as manual means, traction, and mobilization; in cases where dysfunction persists or is recurrent and in any cases at sites of persistent strain and pain in fascia or ligament, refurbishing of the collagen fibers should be attempted.

Prolotherapy

That the provocation of regrowth of connective tissue is possible through stimulating the body cannot be denied. Every surgeon expects this phenomenon to provide healing in sutured wounds. Is it possible to provoke connective tissue fibroblasts into hypertrophy and effect healing, through the laying down of new collagen, without actually cutting them? An inflammation can be *brought to* the relevant site with a needle. A knife is not necessary.

The art of provoking a scar at these sites by searing was first described two and a half millennia ago by Hippocrates[13] and is believed to remain in use in primitive societies. Hippocrates describes the insertion of searing needles into the anterior capsule of the shoulder to stabilize shoulders in javelin throwers, the warriors of Sparta. Interestingly, shoulder instability among contemporary athletes still responds to proliferant therapy. However, searing is no longer necessary; various chemical irritants can be injected through a hollow needle to the appropriate site.

The modern use of sclerotherapy hails to the herniologists of a century and a half ago, an era that antedates antiseptic surgery. In 1837, Valpeau of Paris described the use of scar formation in hernias for their repair.

Earl Gedney, an osteopath from Philadelphia familiar with the sclerosing techniques of herniologists and venologists, was the first to introduce injection techniques for ligaments in 1937.[10] Gedney injected a "hypermobile sacroiliac joint" first and achieved salutary results. The genealogy of herniology, and later the management of hydroceles and a variety of vein sclerosis techniques, was reviewed extensively in 1939 by Yeomans,[25] and the tradition of vein sclerosis persists today.

The term *sclerotherapy* continued to be used for about two decades until the mid 1950s when George Hackett, MD, an industrial surgeon from the Midwest, introduced the concept that the hypertrophy of ligamentous tissue might be achieved successfully without necessarily provoking scars and postulated that through fine tuning the amount of inflammation it might be possible to achieve that exact result. To describe this phenomenon, he introduced the term *prolotherapy*, evaluated its benefit in an initial series of studies, and published a number of articles about his experiences. This culminated in a short textbook, the third edition of which was published in 1958,[12] and the tradition of his textbook continues.[14] Through a process of trial and error that was taken on in other English-speaking countries and, in particular, by M.J. Ongley in New Zealand, a number of substances were found to have the maximal therapeutic yield with minimal risk. The clinical benefits of these techniques are familiar to their users.[6]

REFERENCES

1. Bourdillon JF, Day EA: Spinal Manipulation. 4th ed. London, Heinemann, 1987.
2. Coulter HL: Divided Legacy (in 4 vols). Washington DC, Wehawken Book Co., and Berkeley, CA, North Atlantic Books, 1975–1994.
3. Cyriax J: Manual of Orthopedic Medicine. 2nd ed. London, Butterworth, 1993.
4. Cyriax J: Textbook of Orthopedic Medicine. 8th ed. Philadelphia, WB Saunders, 1982.
5. Division of Labor, Statistics and Research: Statistical information from 1988 California Work Injuries and Illnesses. San Francisco, Dept. of Industrial Relations, Division of Labor, Statistics and Research, 1988.
6. Dorman T, Ravin T: Diagnosis and Injection Techniques in Orthopedic Medicine. Baltimore, Williams & Wilkins, 1991.
7. Erasistratos: Galen's System of Philosophy and Medicine (RE Siegel, trans.). New York, Krager, 1968.
8. Flexner A: Medical Education in the United States and Canada. A report to the Carnegie Foundation for the Advancement of Teaching, 1910. The Carnegie Foundation.
9. Fuller RB: World Game Lecture Series. Philadelphia, University of Pennsylvania Museum, 1975.
10. Gedney EH: Hypermobile joint. Osteopathic Profession 4:30–31, 1937.
11. Greenman PE: Principles of Manual Medicine. Baltimore, Williams & Wilkins, 1989.
12. Hackett GS: Ligament and Tendon Relaxation Treated by Prolotherapy. 3rd ed. Springfield, IL, Charles C. Thomas, 1958.
13. Hippocrates: The genuine works of Hippocrates. (Francis Adams, trans.). Baltimore, Williams & Wilkins, 1946.
14. Institute in Basic Life Principles (G. Hemwall), Box 1, Oak Brook, IL 60522-3001.
15. Lovejoy CO, Meindl RS, Pryzbeck TR, Mensforth RP: Chronological metamorphosis of the auricular surface of the ilium: A new method for the determination of adult skeleltal age at death. Am J Phys Anthrop 68:15–28, 1985.
16. Mennell J: Back Pain. Boston, Little, Brown & Co., 1960.
17. Mennell J: The Science and Art of Joint Manipulation. London, Churchill, 1952.
18. Ongley MJ, Klein RG, Dorman TA, et al: A new approach to the treatment of chronic back pain. Lancet 2:143–146, 1987.
19. Peikoff L: The analytic-synthetic dichotomy. In Rand A: Introduction to Objectivist Epistemology. New York, Nal Books, 1979, pp 88–127.
20. Popper KR: The Logic of Scientific Discovery. Harper & Row, 1959 (Translation of original German text, 1934).
21. Praxagoras, FR. 16 K V 105 through 106 and 46 K XIV 698 as quoted in Coulter HL: Divided Legacy. Vol 1. Washington DC, Wehawken Book Co., 1975.
22. Stevens A: Side bending and axial rotation of the sacrum inside the pelvic girdle. Proceedings of the First International Congress on Low Back Pain and the Sacroiliac Joint. San Diego, November 1990.
23. Still AT: The Philosophy and Mechanical Priciples of Osteopathy. Kansas City, MO, Hudson-Kimberly Publishing, 1892.
24. Vleeming, Volkers AC, Snijders CJ, Stoeckart R: Relation between form and function in the sacroiliac joint. Part II: Biomechanical aspects. Spine 15:133–136, 1990.
25. Yeomans FC (ed): Sclerosing Therapy, the Injection Treatment of Hernia, Hydrocele, Varicose Veins and Hemorrhoids. Baltimore, Williams & Wilkins, 1939.

F. H. WILLARD, PhD

THE ANATOMY OF THE LUMBOSACRAL CONNECTION

From the Department of Anatomy
University of New England
Biddeford, Maine
and
The European School of
  Osteopathy
Maidstone, Kent
England

Reprint requests to:
F. H. Willard, PhD
Department of Anatomy
University of New England
11 Hills Beach Road
Biddeford, ME 04005

The lumbosacral region contains five lumbar vertebrae, the sacrum and two innominate bones articulated by surrounding connective-tissue components. Although described as separate entities in most textbooks of anatomy, the soft-tissue, fibrous structures of the lumbosacral region form a continuous ligamentous stocking into which the lumbar vertebrae and sacrum are positioned. The muscles that represent the prime movers in the lumbosacral region, such as the multifidus, gluteus maximus, and biceps femoris, have various attachments to this elongated, ligamentous stocking. The muscular and ligamentous relationships composing the lumbosacral connection are of extreme importance in stabilizing the lumbar vertebrae and sacrum during the transfer of energy from the upper body to the lower extremities. This arrangement has been termed a self-bracing mechanism;[55] as such, its dysfunction is critical to failure of the lower back.

A critical relationship also exists between the neural components of the lumbosacral region and the surrounding ligamentous structures. Current research, using immunohistochemical techniques to identify specific types of axons, suggests that all of these connective tissue structures receive a supply of small-caliber, primary afferent fibers, typical of nerves involved in nociception. Irritation of primary afferent nociceptive axons initiates the release of neuropeptides that interact with fibroblasts, mast cells, and immune cells in the surrounding connective tissue.[36] The resultant cascade of events, referred to as a neurogenic inflammatory response, is thought to play a major role in degenerative diseases and prolon-

SPINE: State of the Art Reviews—Vol. 9, No. 2, May 1995
Philadelphia, Hanley & Belfus, Inc.

333

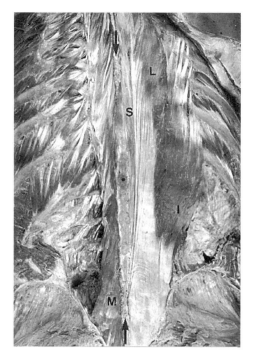

FIGURE 1. The three lumbar paravertebral muscles. The right side illustrates the iliocostalis muscle (I) laterally and the longissimus muscle (L) medially. The left side reveals a deeper dissection illustrating the multifidus muscle (M). Arrows top and bottom are aligned along the spinous processes of the thoracic and lumbar vertebrae (midline). The thicker multifidus muscle is seen differentiating into the thin, flattened semispinalis muscle at the superior end of the lumbar vertebral column (asterisk).

gation of low back pain.[18,30,62,63] This chapter examines recent advances in understanding of the lumbosacral region structure and its innervation.

LIGAMENTOUS STRUCTURE OF THE LUMBAR REGION

The various ligaments of the lumbar vertebral column form a continuous, dense stocking of connective tissue that surrounds the vertebrae and extends into the sacral area. For ease of description, the components of the vertebral connective-tissue sheath are discussed in three parts: the ligaments of the neural arch, the capsule of the facet joints, and the ligaments of the vertebral body. The three divisions, however, are for convenience only; in reality, the connective-tissue components are all continuous across the pedicles of the vertebrae.

Neural Arch Ligaments

The neural arch of each lumbar vertebra is composed of the pedicles, laminae, transverse processes, and spine. Two major ligaments surround the neural arch: the ligamentum flavum and the interspinous ligament. Two small ligaments are also present: the supraspinous ligament posteriorly and the intertransverse ligament laterally. To view the ligaments of the neural arch, the multifidus muscle must be removed from the lumbosacral region (Figs. 1 and 2). Although each of these ligaments has a distinct biochemical make-up, they grade together at their boundaries and function as a single unit. To demonstrate this concept, the osseous components of the neural arch were removed with minimal disturbance to the associated ligamentous structures (Figs. 3 and 4). The unitary nature of the supraspinous and intraspinous ligaments and the ligamentum flavum is obvious; they maintain their continuity despite the lack of osseous support.

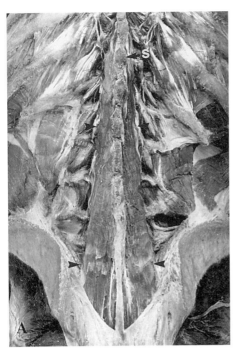 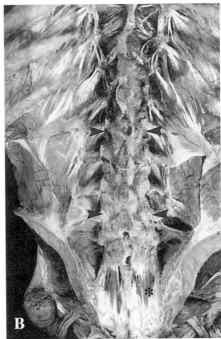

FIGURE 2. The multifidus muscle and its bed. *A*, the pyramidal shaped multifidus muscle is demonstrated between the four arrowheads (S, spinous processes). *B*, the multifidus muscle has been removed to reveal a continuous ligamentous stocking surrounding the neural arch components of the lumbar vertebrae (between arrowheads). On the sacrum, only the deepest laminae of the multifidus remains (asterisk).

The ligamentum flavum, which represents a medial continuation of the articular capsule of the facet joint, stretches between laminae of adjacent vertebra, forming a roof over the spinal canal. Despite a background matrix of collagenous fibers, this ligament has a significantly higher percentage of elastic fibers than surrounding tissue (80% elastic fibers; 20% collagen fibers); hence its yellow color and flexible qualities.[13] The medial fibers of the ligament bridge the gap between the laminae of adjacent vertebra, whereas the lateral fibers attach to the facet joint capsule[7,13,49] (Fig. 3B). The posterior aspect of the medial border of the ligamentum flavum decreases in elastic fiber content and becomes the interspinous ligament. The definitive function for the ligamentum flavum is to provide a roof for the vertebral canal that will not buckle during extension-flexion movements of the vertebral column.[13] The pre-tension in the ligaments at rest (in a neutral position) dissipates as the spinal column is flexed, keeping the ligaments from buckling.[41] The elastic tissue of the ligamentum flavum has no regenerative capacity; thus a damaged ligament is replaced by a cicatrix.[49] In addition, an age-related loss of elastic fibers (and hence of elasticity in the ligamentum flavum) contributes to the progressive loss of tension in the elderly.[41,49]

The interspinous ligament extends between borders of the spines of adjacent vertebrae (Fig. 4). Its anterior border is a continuation of the ligamentum flavum. The posterior border of the interspinous ligament thickens to form the supraspinous

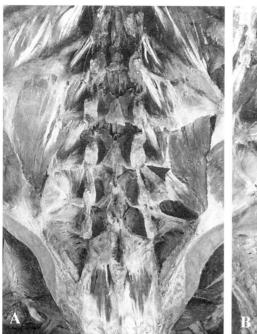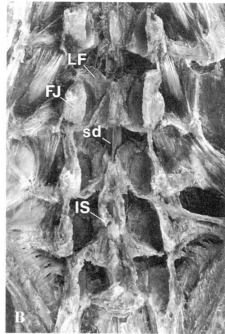

FIGURE 3. The ligamentous stocking of the lumbar vertebrae. *A*, a posterior view of the lumbar spinal column, similar to that in Figure 2, after removing the spinous processes, laminae, and inferior articular processes of the facet joint. *B*, a detailed view of the ligamentous stocking illustrating the ligamentum flavum (LF) extending between the interspinous ligament (IS) medially and the facet joint capsule (FJ) laterally. The arrowhead indicates the same facet joint capsule in both photographs. Between the flaval ligaments, the epidural space and spinal dural (sd) can be seen.

ligament, which, in turn, is anchored to the thoracolumbar fascia. The orientation of fibers in the interspinous ligament has received multiple, conflicting descriptions. In humans, the ligament is best described as a fan (Fig. 5). The narrow or proximal end of the fan blends with the ligamentum flavum and contains elastic fibers,[66] whereas the broad end of the fan extends in a posterior direction toward the tips of the spines and is composed primarily of collagen fibers. In the center of the interspinous ligament the collagen fibers are oriented parallel to the vertebral spines; distally the peripheral collagen fibers flare posterocranially and posterocaudally.[3,23] This fanlike arrangement allows the ligament to expand as the vertebral spines separate during flexion. Although the fibers of the interspinous ligament are described as resisting the separation of the vertebral spines during flexion,[13] the most likely function of the ligament, given the anteroposterior orientation of its fibers, is to act as an anchor, transmitting the anteroposterior pull of the thoracolumbar fascia, into which it is attached via the supraspinous ligament,[23] into an increased tension in the ligamentum flavum. This increased tension would assist in preventing the latter ligament from buckling onto the spinal cord and would also assist in alignment of the lumbar vertebrae. Chondrocytes are present along the osseous borders of the interspinous ligaments, and age-related chondrification begins after the third decade of life.[66] Degenerative

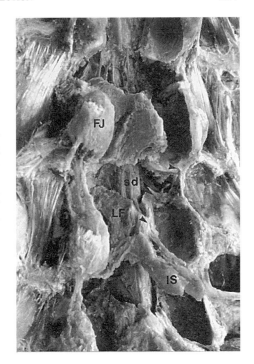

FIGURE 4. A side view of the lumbar ligamentous stocking. The facet joint marked FJ is the same as that marked FJ in Figure 3A. The continuity of the flaval ligament (LF) with the facet joint capsule and interspinous ligament (IS) is indicated by the arrowheads. The spinal dura (sd) can be seen in the epidural space.

processes in the motion segment of the vertebrae appear to enhance chondrification of the interspinous ligament. All of these events affecting the interspinous ligament should diminish the ability of the thoracolumbar fascia to influence the alignment of the lumbar vertebra and thereby increase their risk of destructive injury.

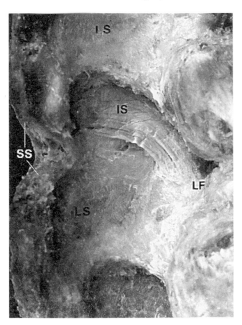

FIGURE 5. A magnified view of the interspinous ligament (top is superior, left is posterior). The lumbar spinous processes (LS) are superior and inferior to the ligament. Note the fanlike orientation of the collagenous fibers in the ligament. The proximal end of the ligament is continuous with the ligamentum flavum (LF), and the distal end of the ligament is embedded in the supraspinous ligament (SS). This latter structure is attached to the thoracolumbar fascia. This arrangement would transform any increased tension in the thoracolumbar fascia into increased tension on the ligamentum flavum, resulting in an alignment of the lumbar vertebra.

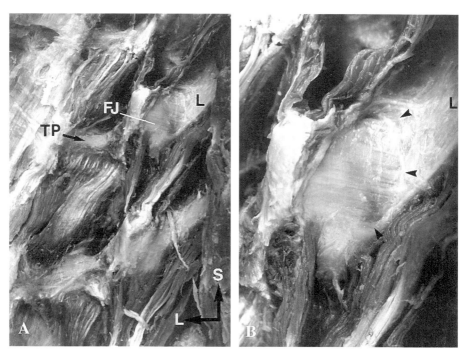

FIGURE 6. The facet joint capsule. *A*, a dorsal view of the lumbar spinal column with all but the deepest laminae of the multifidus muscle removed to reveal the facet joint capsule (FJ), vertebral laminae (L), and transverse processes (TP) of a lumbar vertebra. The right side is aligned along the midline of the body. The orientation figure in the lower right indicates superior (S) and lateral (L) directions. *B*, an enlarged view of the lumbar facet joint capsule marked FJ in 6A. The arrowheads mark the medial border of the capsule as it attaches to the vertebral laminae (L). Note the horizontal orientation to the collagenous fibers in the capsule. This orientation is orthogonal to the long axis of the joint. The capsule is strongest on its posterior (current view) and anterior sides and weakest superiorly and inferiorly.

Of the two small ligaments associated with the neural arch, the supraspinous ligament is the more prominent. It forms the posterior border of the interspinous ligament and fuses with the overlying thoracolumbar fascia. In this position the interspinous and supraspinous ligaments act as force transducers, translating the tension of the thoracolumbar fascia to the lumbar vertebrae. The supraspinous ligament becomes progressively less organized and in some individuals may not extend caudal to L4.[13] It often presents with fatty involution late in life.[21] Finally, the small intertransverse ligament arises from the periosteal tissue surrounding the transverse processes and pedicle of the lumbar vertebrae. Caudally, this tissue expands to represent the iliolumbar ligament.

Articular Capsular Ligament

The lumbar facet or zygapophoseal joints consist of two opposed and vertically oriented plates surrounded by a fibrous capsule.[44] These joints contain a true synovial space, synovial membrane, and associated fluid. The joint capsule represents a connective-tissue bridge between the ligaments of the neural arch and the ligaments of the vertebral body. It is composed of dense connective tissue in which the predominant orientation of the collagenous fibers is orthagonal to the joint line (the plane on which the two facet plates oppose each other; Fig. 6). The capsule is bound tightly to the articular processes with the exception of the inferior and superior recesses, each of which consists of a loosened fold in the capsule wall. This arrangement allows a gliding movement in the sagittal plane but restricts range of motion in the horizontal plane. Each recess has a small defect that is capable of transmitting fat from the capsular space outward.[13] The capsule is reinforced dorsally by the multifidus muscle and ventrally by the ligamentum flavum. It is weakest around the superior recess, which may burst from effusion during arthrography.[16] The inferior border of the capsule is continuous with the ligamentum flavum, the medial border with the periosteum of the lamina, and the lateral border with the periosteum of the pedicle and vertebral body.

Ligaments Ventral to the Facet Joints

The vertebral bodies are surrounded by a well-developed periosteum. This sheath may be envisioned as a dense stocking of connective tissue that houses the vertebrae and the annular ligaments of the intervertebral disks. Dorsally, the periosteum of the vertebral body is continuous with that of the pedicles and laminae. Embedded in the periosteal sheath of the vertebrae are two longitudinal thickenings: The anterior longitudinal ligament and the posterior longitudinal ligament.

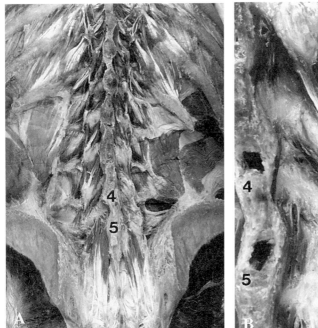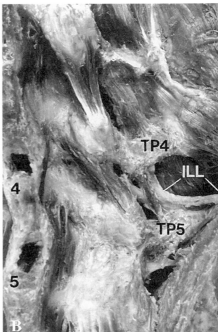

FIGURE 7. A dorsal view of the sacroiliac joint. *A*, the multifidus muscle, except for its deepest laminae, has been removed. The spinous processes of lumbar vertebrae 4 and 5 are indicated. *B*, an enlarged view of the iliolumbar ligament (ILL) from 7A. The ligament attaches to the transverse processes of lumbar vertebrae 4 and 5 (TP4 and TP5). The spinous processes of lumbar vertebrae 4 and 5 are indicated.

The anterior longitudinal ligament consists of a thickened band of vertically oriented collagenous fibers that extends from the cervical region into the sacrum, where it is continuous with the anteromedial aspect of the sacroiliac joint capsule.[13] The deepest bands of collagenous fibers are the shortest and extend from one vertebral body to the next, bridging the annular ligament of the intervertebral disk. The more superficial bands of the ligament span longer distances. In the lumbar region, the anterior longitudinal ligament serves as an attachment for the crura of the diaphragm. Although the main attachments of the crura are in the region of the upper three lumbar vertebrae, some of the crural fibers extend to the lower lumbar region.

The posterior longitudinal ligament is also embedded in the periosteum of the vertebrae and extends from the cervical region to the periosteum of the sacrum.[13] As the ligament descends along the anterior wall of the vertebral canal, it narrows to pass around the bases of the pedicles and expands over the annular ligament of the intervertebral disks. This undulation imparts a serrated appearance to the longitudinal profile of the ligament. The posterior longitudinal ligament is much thinner, both in width and thickness, than its anterior counterpart; the main opposition to flexion of the lumbar spine therefore comes from the ligamentum flavum.[64]

The two longitudinal ligaments and the ligamentum flavum stabilize the lumbar vertebral column in flexion (posterior longitudinal ligament and ligamentum flavum) and extension (anterior longitudinal ligament). The ligaments are most vulnerable to injury when in rotation, especially the anterior longitudinal ligament.[51] Of particular interest is the observation that data on load-deformation values for the anterior longitudinal ligament are similar to data obtained from the ligamentum flavum, suggesting that the two major stabilizing ligaments are balanced in their design.[43] The anterior longitudinal ligament has also been demonstrated to suffer significant age-related decreases in biomechanical parameters.[43]

LIGAMENTS OF THE SACRAL REGION

Iliolumbar Ligament

The iliolumbar ligament is a complex structure that extends from the transverse processes of the lower two lumbar vertebrae to the ileal crest and blends with the interosseous ligaments of the sacroiliac joint (Fig. 7). It has received numerous and varied descriptions. Williams et al.[65] describe superior and inferior bands in the ligament; the inferior band is called the lumbosacral ligament. Kapandji[27] describes superior and inferior bands with an occasional sacral band below the inferior band; O'Rahilly[42] describes anterior, superior, and inferior bands; and Bogduk and Twomey[13] describe anterior, posterior, superior, inferior, and vertical iliolumbar divisions. A recent study based on 100 specimens reported only two parts to the ligament: anterior and posterior.[20] My experience is that the individual bands of fascia are highly variable in number and form but consistently blend superiorly with the intertransverse ligaments of the lumbar vertebrae and inferiorly with the sacroiliac ligaments. The iliolumbar ligament arises from the transverse processes of L5 vertebrae as well as from the transverse processes of L4 and L5 in some individuals (Figs. 7 and 8), contrary to the observations of Hanson and Sonesson.[20] The iliolumbar ligament was previously described as developing from the inferior border of the quadratus lumborum muscle in the second decade of life.[37] However, this theory recently was refuted by observation of the ligament in the fetus as early as gestational ages 11–15 weeks,[57] a finding verified by Hanson and Sonesson.[20] The iliolumbar ligament is subject to fatty degeneration after the sixth decade of life. The major

FIGURE 8. A dorsal view of the sacroiliac joint. *A,* the multifidus muscle has been entirely removed to reveal the interosseous ligaments of the sacroiliac joint. The long posterior sacroiliac ligament (LPSIL), the facet joint between the 4th and 5th lumbar vertebra (4/5), and the sacrotuberous ligament (ST) are indicated as landmarks. *B,* an enlarged view of the sacroiliac joint showing the interosseious ligaments (IOL), the facet joint between the 4th and 5th lumbar vertebrae (4/5), and the iliolumbar ligaments (ILL). The iliolumbar ligament is seen attaching to the transverse processes of L4 and L5. Each process is located opposite the facet joint capsule marked with an asterisk.

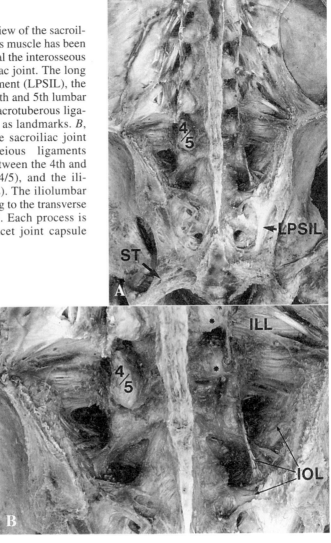

function of the ligament is to restrict motion at the lumbosacral junction, particularly sidebending. After bilateral transection of the iliolumbar ligament, rotation about the vertebral axis increased by 18%, extension by 20%, flexion by 23%, and lateral bending by 29%.[67] Thus, the iliolumbar ligament represents a critical structure for stabilizing the lumbar vertebrae on the sacral base.

Articular Capsule of the Sacroiliac Joint

At the caudal end of the lumbar ligaments lies the capsular structure surrounding the sacroiliac joint (Figs. 8 and 9). This joint is synovial, with a C-shaped articular

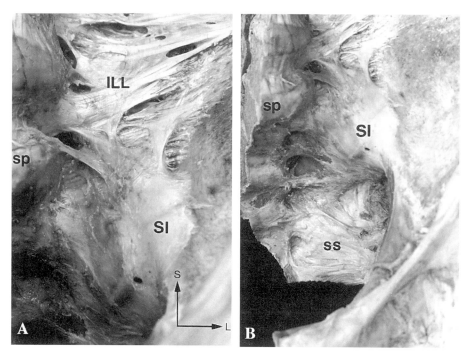

FIGURE 9.   An anterior view of the sacroiliac joint: the pelvic basin after removal of all of the pelvic contents and endopelvic fascia. *A,* the superior portion of the sacroiliac joint (SI) demonstrating its smooth surface and its continuity with the iliolumbar ligament (ILL). *B,* the inferior portion of the sacroiliac joint (SI) demonstrating its continuity with the sacrospinous ligament (SS). In *A* and *B,* the sacral promontory (SP) is marked for reference. Superior (S) and lateral (L) directions are indicated in A.

surface; the longer limb of the joint is oriented posteriorly and the shorter limb superiorly. Range of motion is limited.[60,64] Its anatomy and development were reviewed by Bernard and Cassidy.[8] The joint surface is derived, in part, from the first three sacral vertebrae; its sacral surface is lined with hyaline cartilage and its ileal surface with fibrocartilage (Fig. 10). The joint is surrounded by a tough capsule with several remarkably different surfaces (see Figs. 8 and 9). The superior aspect of the joint capsule is a caudal extension of the iliolumbar ligament. The anterior aspect is composed of a smooth sheet of dense connective tissue stretched between the ventral surfaces of the sacral alar and ilium. The caudal border of the anterior sacroiliac capsule blends with the rostral edge of the sacrospinous ligament. The posterior aspect of the joint capsule is much more complex than its anterior counterpart; it consists of numerous, discontinuous interwoven bands of dense connective tissue. The short interosseous sacroiliac ligaments arise on the intermediate and lateral sacral crest and attach to the rough sacropelvic surface of the ilium. The long interosseous sacroiliac ligaments extend from the median sacral crest, diagonal in a superior direction across the sacral gutter, and attach to the posterior superior spine of the ilium. Several other pelvic structures anchor into the posterior interosseous ligaments of the sacroiliac joint. The sacrotuberous ligament attaches to the long interosseous ligaments of

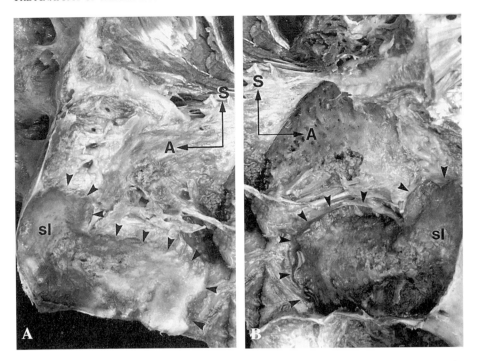

FIGURE 10. The internal features of the sacroiliac joint. The sacroiliac joint seen in Figure 9 was opened to display its medial (*A*) and lateral (*B*) surfaces. The boundaries of the joint are marked with arrowheads. The anterior boundary is formed by a precise capsule, the posterior boundary is formed by the interweaving of the interosseous ligaments. The joint has a superior limb (sl) and inferior limb. The orientation arrows indicate the superior (S) and anterior (A) directions. The medial surface is concave and covered with hyaline cartilage with associated fatty deposits; the lateral surface is convex and covered with fibrocartilage.

the joint capsule laterally, and the thoracolumbar fascia anchors to the same interosseous ligaments posteriorly. The anchoring portion of the thoracolumbar fascia also forms a prominent raphe separating the multifidus and gluteus maximus muscles (see Fig. 12).

The articular surfaces of the sacroiliac joint are smooth and flattened at birth, and the long axis of the joint is oriented parallel to that of the lumbar spine[8] (Fig. 10). The joint is remodeled during puberty into the adult C-shaped orientation with roughened surface. The ileal surface, lined with fibrocartilage, develops a crescent-shaped ridge along its long axis (Fig. 10A), whereas the sacral surface, lined with hyaline cartilage, forms a concavity complementary to the convexity of the ileal surface in the second decade of life (Fig. 10B). These changes in the surface of the joint contribute to its stability and limited range of motion.[54] Thus the interlocking surfaces of the joint form the centerpiece in the self-bracing model of sacroiliac joint function.[55] A series of age-related degenerative changes affect the joint, especially after fifth decade of life. The cartilagenous surfaces begin to degenerate, with ossification between the two articular surfaces, especially in men.[8] Such changes eventually restrict motion of the joint even further.

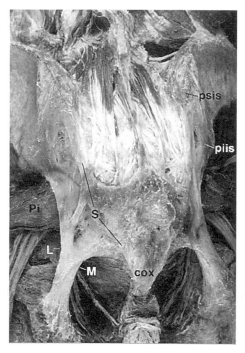

FIGURE 11. A dorsal view of the sacroiliac joint and sacrotuberous ligament. All but the deepest laminae of the multifidus muscle (M) have been removed. The sacrotuberous ligaments stretch from the ischial tuberosity (it) to the coccyx (cox) medially and the posterior ileal spines superolaterally. The posterior superior ileal spine (psis) and the posterior inferior ileal spine (piis) are marked on the contralateral side. Three major bands of the ligament are seen: lateral (L), medial (M), and superior (S). The lateral band spans the pyriformis muscle (Pi) to reach the ilium inferior to the posterior inferior ileal spine (piis). The medial band attaches to the coccyx, and the superior band courses superficial to the posterior long interosseous ligament to connect the coccyx with the posterior ileal spines. Tendons of the multifidus pass between the superior band and the posterior long interosseous ligament to insert into the body of the sacrotuberous ligament.

Sacrotuberous Ligament

The sacrotuberous ligament is in fact a specialization of the posteroinferior aspect of the sacroiliac joint capsule. It is a triangular-shaped structure extending between the posterior ileal spines, sacroiliac joint capsule, coccygeal vertebrae, and ischial tuberosity (Fig. 11). The tendon of the biceps femoris often reaches over the tuberosity to attach to the sacrotuberous ligament,[59] and an occasional aberrant muscle derived from the biceps femoris attaches its entire superior head to this ligament.[2] The tendons of the deepest laminae of the multifidus often extend into the sacrotuberous ligament from its superior surface (see Fig. 11). The ligament can be divided into three large fibrous bands. Its prominent lateral band reaches from the posteroinferior ileal spine to the ischial tuberosity, and its medial band connects the coccygeal vertebrae with the ischial tuberosity. The superior band is the thinnest and forms a plate stretching between the posterior ileal spines and the coccygeal vertebrae. Along its medial edge, the superior band merges with the interosseous ligaments of the sacroiliac joint capsule. The body of the sacrotuberous ligament is made from the fusion of these bands and occasionally is penetrated by branches from the gluteal neurovascular bundle.

Sacrospinous Ligament

The sacrospinous ligament is in fact a specialization of the anteroinferior aspect of the sacroiliac joint capsule. It is a triangular-shaped structure (see Fig. 9B) arising from the coccygeal vertebrae and inferior aspect of the sacroiliac joint capsule. Its distal attachment is to the spine of the ischium. Proximally, most of its fibers blend with those of the sacroiliac joint capsule. The ligament forms the posterolateral border of the pelvic outlet and has been used as an anchor into which the pelvic floor may be secured in patients with eversion of the vagina.[40,47]

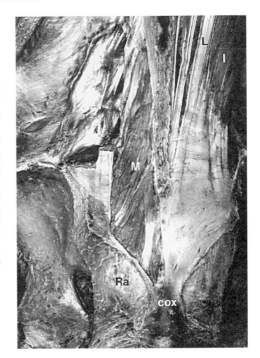

FIGURE 12. A dorsal view of the sacroiliac region with the gluteus maximus muscle removed. The tendinous insertion of the iliocostalis (I) and longissimus (L) muscles has been opened to expose the multifidus muscle (M). The raphe (Ra) separating the multifidus and gluteus muscles stretches from the coccyx (cox) to the posterior superior ileal spine (asterisk). Its anterior border is blended with the sacroiliac joint capsule and its posterior border is blended with the thoracolumbar fascia. The rough surface visible on this raphe represents the attachment site for the gluteal muscle.

Summary

The ligamentous structures of the lumbosacral connection form a continuous stocking of dense connective tissue that houses the lumbar vertebrae and sacrum and provides attachment sites for associated muscles. This complicated ligamentous structure plays a key role in the self-bracing mechanism of the pelvis, a mechanism that maintains the integrity of the low back and pelvis during transfer of energy from the spine to the lower extremities.[59,61] Unilateral lesions of the ligaments surrounding the sacroiliac joint increase the range of motion (and hence decrease the stability) of the joint under compressive loads.[54] The ligamentous mechanism of the lumbosacral region is influenced by several major muscle groups in the low back and pelvis, each of which is discussed below.

MAJOR MUSCLE GROUPS ASSOCIATED WITH LUMBOSACRAL LIGAMENTOUS STRUCTURES

Multifidus Muscle

The paravertebral muscles in the lumbar region include three large muscles, each in its own fascial compartment and arranged from lateral to medial: the iliocostalis, longissimus, and multifidus[10] (see Fig. 1). The two lateral muscles—the iliocostalis and longissimus—arise from the ileal crest and thoracolumbar fascia but, with the exception of a few medial slips from the longissimus, do not attach to the lumbar vertebrae. The multifidus has major attachments to the spinous process, interspinous ligaments, laminae, and articular capsules of the lumbar vertebrae as well as to the medial, intermediate, and lateral sacral crests, sacropelvic surface of the ilium, and thoracolumbar fascia. The attachment of the muscles to the thoracolumbar fascia represents a raphe separating the multifidus from the gluteus maximus muscle (Fig. 12). The anterior border of the raphe is anchored in the sacroiliac joint capsule, and the posterior border of the raphe becomes part of the thoracolumbar fascia. Finally, tendinous slips of the multifidus muscle pass under the long posterior interosseous ligaments to join with the sacrotuberous ligament. These connections integrate the multifidus into the ligamentous support system of the sacroiliac joint.

The fibers of the multifidus are aligned in the vertical plane with only slight horizontal deviations. This arrangement is superior for movement in the sagittal plane, making the multifidus the main extensor muscle for the lumbar spine.[38] However, due to its geometry, the multifidus is capable of only slight movements in the horizontal plane. The long fibers in the body of the muscle span multiple segments, thus giving the multifidus muscle its additional role as a prime stabilizer of the lumbar spine[15,38] Finally, by increasing tension on the thoracolumbar fascia, sacroiliac ligaments, and sacrotuberous ligaments, activation of the multifidus also contributes to the self-bracing mechanism of the pelvis and to the transfer of energy from the upper body to the lower extremities.

Latissimus Dorsi Muscle

The upper extremity is anchored to the body through an anterior muscular hood (the pectoral muscles) and a posterior muscular hood (the latissimus dorsi). The latissimus dorsi has its axial attachment to the thoracolumbar fascia, ileal crest, and three or four caudal ribs. Its appendicular attachment is to the intertubecular groove of the humerus. This arrangement allows the activation of the latissimus dorsi, expressed through the thoracolumbar fascia, to influence the supraspinous and interspinous ligaments and the spines in the lumbar region. Through the action of this muscle, expressed via the thoracolumbar fascia, the upper extremity can assist the lower extremity during locomotion.

Gluteus Maximus Muscle

The gluteus maximus is the largest muscle of the body. It is attached to the posterior surface of the ileal blade and crest, the thoracolumbar fascia and its associated raphe (which also functions as an attachment for the multifidus), the sacrotuberous ligament, and the lateral crest of the sacrum and coccygeal vertebrae. Its appendicular attachment involves the iliotibial band and the gluteal tuberosity of the femur. Through its attachment to the raphe of the thoracolumbar fascia, the gluteus maximus is also opposed to the ipsilateral multifidus muscle and, most likely, coupled to the contralateral latissimus dorsi muscle.[58] Thus, through its attachments to the ligaments and fascia of the sacroiliac joint, the gluteus maximus muscle becomes a major contributing force to the self-bracing mechanism of the pelvis.[55]

Biceps Femoris Muscle (Long Head)

The long head of the biceps femoris muscle reaches over the posterior surface of the ischial tuberosity to attach to the sacrotuberous ligament.[59] Its inferior attachment is to the lateral aspect of the fibular head, lateral condyle of the tibia, and a sheet of fascia covering the lateral aspect of the leg. Thus, the biceps femoris represents a continuum from the sacroiliac ligaments to the fibula and investing fascia of the leg. Contraction of the biceps femoris extends the thigh and pulls the sacrum against the ilium, tightening the sacroiliac joint. As such it contributes to the self-bracing mechanism in the pelvis and helps to stabilize the sacroiliac joint during the force of transfer from spine to lower extremity.[59]

Piriformis Muscle

Inside the pelvic basin, the piriformis muscle influences the integrity of the sacroiliac joint. Proximally, the piriformis muscle attaches to the sacrum, sacro-tuberous ligament, margin of the greater sciatic foramen, and medial edge of the sacroiliac joint capsule. Distally, the muscle reaches out through the greater sciatic foramen to attach to the greater trochanter of the femur. Contraction of the piriformis rotates the thigh laterally, stabilizes the head of the femur in the acetabulum, and places tension on the sacroiliac joint capsule, pulling the sacrum against the ilium and thereby contributing to the self-bracing mechanism.[59]

Summary

The ligamentous stocking of the lumbar spine and sacroiliac joint capsule fuse to the anterior surface of the thoracolumbar fascia. In turn, this large sheet of fascia and the lumbosacral ligaments serve as attachment sites for the major prime movers and stabilizing muscles of the spine. Activation of these muscles helps to tighten the connective-tissue support structures, thereby stabilizing the lumbosacral spine and by contributing to the self-bracing mechanism.[55] In addition, large muscles of the extremities, such as the latissimus dorsi and the gluteus maximus, attach to the borders of the thoracolumbar fascia. This arrangement facilitates the transfer of energy from the upper extremities, through the spine, and into the lower extremities. The close coupling of muscles through the thoracolumbar fascia and the attachments to the ligamentous stocking of the spine allow motion in the upper limbs to assist in rotation of the trunk and movement of the lower extremities in gait. Thus an integrated system is created.[58]

INNERVATION OF THE LUMBOSACRAL REGION

The ligaments of the lumbosacral region are innervated predominantly with small-caliber primary afferent fibers and sympathetic efferent fibers. Such fibers are typical of those involved with the detection of nociception and initiation of inflammatory processes. Thus, the nerve supply to the lumbosacral ligaments plays a key role in the integrity of this region. The tissue of the lumbosacral region has three separate sources of innervation: the dorsal rami of the spinal nerves, sinu vertebral nerve (or recurrent meningeal nerve), and somatosympathetic nerves. Each nerve supply covers a different area of tissue and, based on distribution, creates a different pattern of pain perception when irritated.

Lumbosacral Dorsal Rami

The dorsal ramus leaves the spinal nerve as the nerves exit the lumbar intervertebral canals. As the nerve wraps around the facet joint directly below, it divides into three main branches: the lateral branch, which innervates the lateral fascial compartment containing the iliocostalis muscle; the intermediate branch, which innervates the intermediate fascial compartment containing the longissimus muscle; and the medial branch, which innervates the medial fascial compartment containing the multifidus muscle as well as the ligaments and intrinsic muscles of the lumbar and sacral vertebrae[11] (Fig. 13). Specifically, the medial compartment contains three major muscles (multifidus, interspinalis, and intertransversarii medialis) as well as skeletal elements, such as the interspinous ligament, facet joints, and ligament flavum. Inferiorly, the dorsal and ventral rami of L5 and of the sacral roots innervate the sacroiliac joint capsule.[24] Irritation of the small-caliber, primary afferent fibers of the dorsal ramus innervating these tissue results in perception of pain. This pain is

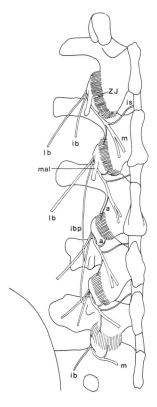

FIGURE 13. A dorsal view of the lumbar spine illustrating the three major branches of the dorsal ramus. (a, articular twigs from medial branch; ib, intermediate branch; ibp, intermediate branch plexus; is, interspinous twig from medial branch; lb, lateral branch; m, medial medial branch; mal, mamillio-accessory ligament; ZJ, zygoapophyseal joint. (From Bogduk N: The innervation of the lumbar spine. Spine 8:286–293, 1983; with permission.)

usually sharp and burning, like spinal root pain, and may refer to the area supplied by the corresponding ventral ramus, thus mimicking sciatica. Because the dorsal ramus also innervates muscle groups in the back, compression or damage to this nerve may present with signs of denervation weakness as well as with pain.

Sinu Vertebral or Recurrent Meningeal Nerves

Before its division into dorsal and ventral rami, the spinal nerve gives off a small branch that recurves into the intervertebral foramen to reach the vertebral canal (Fig. 14). The terminal branches service the posterior longitudinal ligament, periosteum on the posterior aspect of the vertebral body, outer layers of the intervertebral disks, and anterior surface of the spinal dura.[11,19,56] In an elegant study of the sinu vertebral nerve, Groen and colleagues[19] demonstrated that it may travel up and/or down the vertebral canal at least 2–3 segments from the point of entry (Fig. 14, A–F). In addition, it may cross the midline to innervate tissue on the contralateral side (Fig. 14D, G, H). Of note, some fibers of the sinu vertebral nerve cross the vertebral canal and subsequently pass outward through the contralateral intervertebral foramina (Fig. 14H).

Based on this pattern of innervation, irritation of the small-caliber, primary afferent fibers in the sinu vertebral nerve may refer pain several segments up or down the spinal cord as well as to the contralateral side of the body. In addition, slight movements of any obstacle in the vertebral canal or intervertebral foramina may irritate sinu vertebral fibers from either left or right or both sides of the body. This

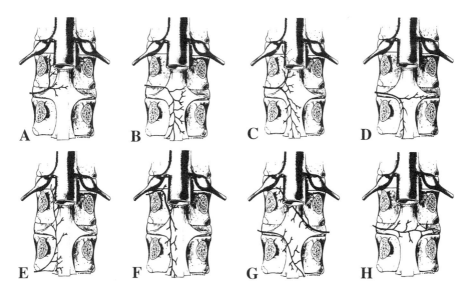

FIGURE 14. Eight variations in the distribution of the sinu vertebral nerve. (From Groen GJ, Baljet B, Drukker J: Nerves and nerve plexuses of the human vertebral column. Am J Anat 188:282–296, 1990; with permission.)

arrangement also offers a possible explanation for the shifting of pain patterns from side to side in a given patient. Finally, because the sinu vertebral nerve does not supply any skeletal muscle, compression or other damage does not present with signs of denervation weakness.

Somatosympathetic Nerves

No somatic nerves (direct branches of the dorsal or ventral rami or spinal nerves) reach the anterior aspect of the vertebral bodies. However, this area is serviced by sensory fibers travelling in branches of the sympathetic trunk.[11,19,56] These small-caliber, primary afferent fibers wrap around the anterior longitudinal ligament and the periosteum on the anterior aspect of the vertebral body and reach into the outer layers of the intervertebral disks (Fig. 15). To return to the spinal cord, the sensory fibers follow the sympathetic trunk. At least some of these fibers are capable of using only white rami to gain access to the spinal nerve and dorsal root ganglia. Therefore, the sensory fibers pass superiorly in the sympathetic trunk to reach the lowest white rami located at the thoracolumbar junction.[26] Thus, noxious stimuli in the loser lumbar and sacral levels ascend in the sympathetic trunk to present to the spinal cord at the thoracolumbar junction. This circuitous route results in referral of pain and subsequent facilitation of spinal segments in the lower thoracic and upper lumbar region from dysfunction of lumbosacral and pelvic structures.

Noxious stimuli that activate somatosympathetic fibers result in what has been described as a diffuse, dense, boring pain that refers to the zones of Head in the thoracolumbar region.[26] In a study of pain, patients with vertebral lesions involving the anterior territory (anterior longitudinal ligament) described the pain as deep, dense, and hard to localize. In general, referral zones involved upper lumbar segments along the flank of the body and extended downward into the thigh. This pattern was present even in patients with anterior disk lesions as low as L5. The somatosympa-

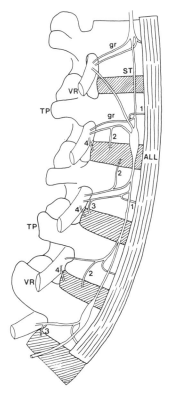

FIGURE 15. A side view of the lumbar spine illustrating the somatosympathetic nerves. The sympathetic trunk communicates with the ventral ramus (VR) through grey rami (gr). Small branches (1) from the sympathetic trunk provide sympathetic efferent and primary afferent fibers to the anterior longitudinal ligament (ALL). Small branches (2 and 3) from the grey rami and ventral ramus (4) reach the intervertebral disk. (TP transverse process). (From Bogduk N: The innervation of the lumbar spine. Spine 8:286–293, 1983; with permission.)

thetic pattern of pain contrasted with the pattern in patients suffering pain from posterior lesions that irritate axons in the sinu vertebral nerve or dorsal ramus. The pain pattern in the latter patients was related more closely to the segment of injury and had a sharp or burning quality. As with the sinu vertebral nerve, the somatosympathetic axons do not supply any skeletal muscle, therefore damage does not present with signs of denervation weakness.

INNERVATION OF SPECIFIC LUMBOSACRAL STRUCTURES

The general innervation patterns described above demonstrate that most structures in the lumbosacral region receive a generous nerve supply. However, a critical question involves the type of axons and terminals in specific connective tissues. The type of nerve fibers determines the function of the tissue as well as its susceptibility to neurogenic inflammatory processes.[4,36,52] Three general categories of innervation are known: large myelinated sensory axons with encapsulated endings, which are involved with discriminative touch and proprioception; small lightly myelinated or unmyelinated sensory axons with naked nerve endings, which are involved in nociception; and small, lightly myelinated efferent axons, which are involved in the autonomic nervous system. Of the latter two types, the small primary afferent axons often contain neuropeptides such as substance P, calcitonin-generated polypeptide, or somatostatin; axons associated with the autonomic nervous system contain norepinephrine (as indicated by presence of tyrosine hydroxylase) and neuropeptide Y. Both types play critical roles in the induction and maintenance of neurogenic inflammatory processes.[4,36]

Neural Arch Ligaments

Immunohistochemical procedures to label and identify axons in connective tissue allow characterization of the innervation of neural arch ligaments, which are serviced by the medial branch of the dorsal ramus. Small-caliber, primary afferent axons from this nerve have been identified in the supraspinous ligament, interspinous ligament, and ligamentum flavum.[50] In addition, such fibers also have been found in the thoracolumbar fascia.[50,66] Frequently these small axons were seen to leave the areas of the blood vessels and to course through the matrix of the surrounding connective tissue. In addition, axons positive for tyrosine hydroxylase and neuropeptide Y (suggesting that they are sympathetic efferent axons) have been described in the interspinous ligaments.[1] Such results demonstrate the presence of both primary afferent nociceptors and sympathetic axons in the neural arch ligaments of the lumbar spine.

Articular Capsule Ligaments

The facet joint is innervated by branches from the medial divisions of the dorsal rami above and below the joint.[12] This observation suggests that inflammatory or degenerative diseases of any facet joint will activate multiple segments in the spinal cord. Neurophysiologic studies of the lumbar facet joints of rabbits have demonstrated the presence of both high-threshold, slow-conducting fibers and low-threshold, fast-conducting fibers.[68] The former are potential nociceptive axons, and the latter are potential proprioceptive axons. Encapsulated nerve endings, suggestive of proprioceptors, have been observed in facet joint capsules.[25] The presence in the joint capsule and synovial plica of small-caliber, primary afferent fibers containing sensory neuropeptides such as substance P and calcitonin gene-related polypeptide has been confirmed in several anatomic studies.[1,6,17] Many of these primary afferent fibers are present in the connective tissue of the joint capsule, separate from the vasculature.[1] In addition, fibers containing tyrosine hydroxylase and neuropeptide Y, markers for sympathetic axons, have been reported in the joint capsule; however, such axons remain close to the vasculature.[1] The presence of small-caliber, primary afferent fibers in the capsule of the facet joints supports the contention that dysfunction of these joints is a source of low back pain.[8,14,39]

Beamen et al.[6] report that small-caliber fibers, positive for the neuropeptide substance P, were also present in the bone and articular cartilage of normal human facet joints but only in very low numbers. However, neuropeptide-containing axons were present in increased quantity in specimens from patients with degenerative diseases of the facet joints. The fibers were found in erosion channels accompanying the vasculature deep into the bone underlying the articular surface. Such observations suggest that normal facet joints may be refractive to pain because of a limited supply of small-caliber fibers under pressure-bearing surfaces and that degenerative joints become painful, in part, because of the increase in nociceptive fibers associated with pressure-bearing surfaces.

Vertebral Body Ligaments

Small, primary afferent axons have been identified in the posterior longitudinal ligament and in the peripheral portion of the annulus fibrosus.[31,32] Axons positive for tyrosine hydroxylase and neuropeptide Y, suggesting that they are sympathetic efferent axons, have been described in the posterior longitudinal ligament, ventral dura, periosteum of the vertebral body, intervertebral disk, and vertebral body, reaching into the marrow cavities.[1]

Sacral Region Ligaments

The sacroiliac joint only recently has become a focus of attention in low back pain studies, and few studies have examined its innervation. Ikeda[24] reports that the anterosuperior aspect of the joint receives twigs from spinal nerve L5 and that the inferior anterior aspect of the joint is supplied by spinal nerve S2 and other sacral nerves. The posterosuperior aspect of the joint is supplied by lateral branches from the 5th lumbar dorsal ramus and the inferoposterior aspect from a plexus of lateral branches from the sacral dorsal rami. These nerves reach the joint capsule and invade the surrounding ligaments. Axons in the nerves to the sacroiliac joint were approximately 0.2–2.5 µm in diameter and thus are well within the range of group IV (C-fibers) and possibly within the smaller end of the group III (A-delta) fibers. Axons of this size are associated with nociception and may be involved in the perception of pain from the sacroiliac joint. The role of the sacroiliac joint in the generation of chronic low back pain has been previously described[5] and recently has received renewed attention.[53] The finding of small-caliber, primary afferent fibers in the joint capsule supports this concept.

Summary

Recent studies of the lumbosacral ligamentous structure using immunohistochemical techniques have provided evidence that many regions, if not the entire connective-tissue stocking, are innervated by small-caliber, primary afferent fibers. Such nerves not only are in a position to supply the spinal cord with nociceptive stimuli but also are typical of the B-afferent neural system[48] that is capable of secreting proinflammatory neuropeptides. Irritation of primary afferent nociceptor fibers and the subsequent release of such peptides as substance P and calcitonin gene-related polypeptide results in the degranulation of mast cells and release of histamine. This biogenic amine promotes vasodilation as well as leukocyte recruitment and proliferation and further irritates primary afferent fibers, thus initiating the release of more substance P.[4] In addition, substance P stimulates macrophages and monocytes to increase phagocytosis; to release proinflammatory compounds, such as thromoboxane and hydrogen peroxide; and to increase production of cytokines, such as interleukin-1.[45,46] The final products are tissue inflammation and edema. This cascade of events, involving neural-immune interactions, typifies the neurogenic inflammatory process.[36,46] In addition to the primary afferent fibers, sympathetic efferent axons have been detected in much of the connective tissue of the lumbosacral spine. A balanced interaction between the two neural systems is thought to be important for the maintenance of normal tissue texture and normal trafficking of cells through the extracellular matrix of the tissue.[22,28,35] Abnormal activity in either or both systems increases the output of neuropeptides and catecholamine and has been associated with increased susceptibility to degenerative connective-tissue diseases.[4,18,28–30,33,34,36] Thus, the activity of the primary afferent nociceptors and sympathetic efferent fiber systems is an important consideration in maintenance of the integrity of the lumbosacral ligamentous structures.

CONCLUSIONS

This chapter examined the anatomy and innervation of the ligamentous stocking that forms the lumbosacral connection. Although the stocking contains numerous regional ligaments, their continuity gives the structure a unitary function. The ligamentous stocking supports the osseous elements of the lumbosacral spine. In turn, the stocking is anchored to the thoracolumbar fascia of the back. This large sheet of aponeurotic fascia serves as an attachment site for the major muscle groups of the spine, abdomen, and two sets of extremities. Through such connections, the thoracolumbar fascia may assist in the transfer of energy from the upper to the lower body, thus minimizing the stress on the lumbosacral spine and facilitate participation of the upper body in lower body motion, forming the integrated system described by Vleeming et al.[58] Not surprisingly, the thoracolumbar fascia contains both small-caliber fibers, which are typical of nociceptors and sympathetic axons, and large-caliber fibers which are typical of mechanoreception and proprioception. Thus, the force transformation through the thoracolumbar fascia may be under the proprioceptive control of neural elements in this tissue.

Most of the component tissues in the ligamentous stocking of the lumbosacral spine are serviced by both primary afferent nociceptor and sympathetic efferent axons. Because of at least three separate sources of small-caliber fibers in the lumbosacral region, each with a differential distribution within the tissues of the back, several different patterns of pain are established. Finally, a possible interactive role for such neural elements in the normal trophic activity of the tissue has been proposed; however, it is also clear that they are instrumental in orchestrating neurogenic inflammatory processes when they become irritated. Thus, the tissues of the lumbosacral connection receive a nerve supply that is capable of sustaining a prolonged inflammatory response, thereby contributing to the progressive breakdown of function in the back.

ACKNOWLEDGMENT

The author thanks Jane Carreiro, DO, for critical discussion and reading of this paper, Suezan Moore for assistance in preparation of the manuscript, and Ralph Thieme for his dissection skills.

REFERENCES

1. Ahmed M, Bjurholm A, Kreicbergs A, et al: Tyrosine hydroxylase and vasoactive intestinal polypeptide-immunoreactive nerve fibers in the vertebral bodies, disc, dura mater, and spinal ligaments of the rat lumbar spine. Spine 18:268–273, 1993.
2. Akita K, Sakamoto H, Sato T: Innervation of an aberrant digastric muscle in the posterior thigh: Stratified relationships between branches of the inferior gluteal nerve. J Anat 181:503–506, 1992.
3. Aspden RM, Bornstein NH, Hukins DWL: Collagen organization in the interspinous ligament and its relationship to tissue function. J Anat 155:141–151, 1987.
4. Basbaum AI, Levine JD: The contributions of the nervous system to inflammation and inflammatory disease. Can J Physiol Pharmacol 69:647–651, 1991.
5. Beal MC: The sacroiliac problem: Review of anatomy, mechanics, and diagnosis. J Am Osteopath Assoc 81:667–679, 1982.
6. Beaman DN, Graziano GP, Glover RA, et al: Substance P innervation of lumbar spine facet joints. Spine 18:1044–1049, 1993.
7. Behrsin JF, Briggs CA: Ligaments of the lumbar spine: A review. Surg Radiol Anat 10:211–219, 1988.
8. Bernard TN, Casidy JD: The sacroiliac joint syndrome: Pathophysiology, diagnosis, and management. In Frymoyer JW (ed): The Adult Spine. New York, Raven Press, 1991, pp 2107–2130.
9. Bernard TN, Kirkaldy-Willis WH: Recognizing specific characteristics of nonspecific low back pain. Clin Orthop 217:266–280, 1987.
10. Bogduk N: A reappraisal of the anatomy of the human lumbar erector spinae. J Anat 131:525–540, 1980.
11. Bogduk N: The innervation of the lumbar spine. Spine 8:286–293, 1983.
12. Bogduk N, Long DM: The anatomy of the so-called "articular nerves" and their relationship to facet denervation in the treatment of low-back pain. J Neurosurg 51:172–177, 1979.
13. Bogduk N, Twomey LT: Clinical Anatomy of the Lumbar Spine. 2nd ed. Melbourne, Churchill Livingstone, 1991.

14. Carette S, Marcoux S, Truchon R, et al: A controlled trial of corticosteroid injections into facet joints for chronic low back pain. N Engl J Med 325:1002–1007, 1991.

15. Crisco JJ, Panjabi MM: The intersegmental and multisegmental muscles of the lumbar spine: A biomechanical model comparing lateral stabilizing potential. Spine 16:793–799, 1991.

16. Dory MA: Arthrography of the lumbar facet joints. Radiology 140:23–27, 1981.

17. El-Bohy AA, Cavanaugh JM, Getchell ML, et al: Localization of substance P and neurofilament immunocreactive fibers in the lumbar facet joint capsule and supraspinous ligament of the rabbit. Brain Res 460:379–382, 1988.

18. Garrett NE, Mapp PI, Cruwys SC, et al: Role of substance P in inflammatory arthritis. Ann Rheum Dis 51:1014–1018, 1992.

19. Groen GJ, Baljet B, Drukker J: Nerves and nerve plexuses of the human vertebral column. Am J Anat 188:282–296, 1990.

20. Hanson P, Sonesson B: The anatomy of the iliolumbar ligament. Arch Phys Med Rehabil 75:1245–1246, 1994.

21. Heylings DJA: Supraspinous and interspinous ligaments of the human lumbar spine. J Anat 125:127–131, 1978.

22. Holzer P: Local effector functions of capsaicin-sensitive sensory nerve endings: Involvement of tachykinins, calcitonin gene-related polypeptide and other neuropeptides. Neuroscience 24:739–768, 1988.

23. Hukins DWL, Kirby MC, Sikoryn TA, et al: Comparison of structure, mechanical properties, and function of lumbar spinal ligaments. Spine 15:787–795, 1990.

24. Ikeda R: Innervation of the sacroiliac joint. Macroscopical and histological studies. Nippon Ika Daigaku Zasshi 58:587–596, 1991.

25. Jackson HC, Winkelmann RK, Bickel WH: Nerve endings in the human lumbar spinal column and related structures. J Bone Joint Surg 48A:1272–1281, 1966.

26. Jinkins JR, Whittemore AR, Bradley WG: The anatomic basis of vertebrogenic pain and the autonomic syndrome associated with lumbar disk extrusion. AJR 152:1277–1289, 1989.

27. Kapandji IA: The Physiology of the Joints. Vol 3. Edinburgh, Churchill Livingstone, 1974.

28. Kidd BL, Cruwys S, Mapp PI, Black DR: Role of the sympathetic nervous system in chronic joint pain and inflammation. Ann Rheum Dis 51:1188–1191, 1992.

29. Kidd BL, Gibson SJ, O'Higgins F, et al: A neurogenic mechanism for symmetrical arthritis. Lancet 1128:1131, 1989.

30. Kidd BL, Mapp PI, Blake DR, et al: Neurogenic influences in arthritis. Ann Rheum Dis 49:649–652, 1990.

31. Konttinen YT, Gronblad M, Hukkanen M, et al: Pain fibers in osteoarthritis: A review. Semin Arthritis Rheum 18:35–40, 1989.

32. Korkala O, Gronblad M, Liesi P, Karaharju E: Immunohistochemical demonstration of nociceptors in the ligamentous structures of the lumbar spine. Spine 10:156–157, 1985.

33. Lam FY, Ferrell WR: Neurogenic component of different models of acute inflammation in the knee joint. Ann Rheum Dis 50:747–751, 1991.

34. Levine J, Collier DH, Basbaum AI, et al: Hypothesis: The nervous system may contribute to the pathophysiology of rheumatoid arthritis. J Rheumatol 12:406–411, 1985.

35. Levine JD, Coderre TJ, Covinsky K, Basbaum AI: Neural influences on synovial mast cell density in rat. J Neurosci Res 26:301–307, 1990.

36. Levine JD, Fields HL, Basbaum AL: Peptides and the primary afferent nociceptor. J Neurosci 13:2273–2286, 1993.

37. Luk KDK, Ho HC, Leong JCY: The iliolumbar ligament: A study of its anatomy development and clinical significance. J Bone Joint Surg 68B:197–200, 1986.

38. Macintosh J, Bogduk N: The biomechanics of the lumbar multifidus. Clin Biomech 1:205–213, 1986.

39. Mooney V, Robertson J: The facet syndrome. Clin Orthop 115:149–156, 1976.

40. Morley GW, DeLancey JOL: Sacrospinous ligament fixation for eversion of the vagina. Am J Obstet Gynecol 158:872–881, 1988.

41. Nachemson A, Evans J: Some mechanical properties of the third lumbar intervertebral ligament (ligamentum flavum). J Biomech 1:211–220, 1968.

42. O'Rahilly R: Anatomy: R Regional Study of Human Structure. 5th ed. Philadelphia, WB Saunders, 1986.

43. Panjabi MM, White AA: Physical properties and functional biomechanics of the spine. In White AA, Panjabi MM (eds): Clinical Biomechanics of the Spine. Philadelphia, JB Lippincott, 1990, pp 1–83.

44. Paris SV: Anatomy as related to function and pain. Orthop Clin North Am 14:475–489, 1983.

45. Payan DG: Substance P: A neuroendocrine-immune modulator. Hosp Pract 24:67–80, 1989.
46. Payan D: The role of neuropeptides in inflammation. In Gallin JI, Goldstein IM, Snyderman R (eds): Inflammation: Basic Principles and Clinical Correlations. New York, Raven Press, 1992.
47. Porges R, Smilen SW: Long-term analysis of the surgical management of pelvic support defects. Am J Obstet Gynecol 171:1518–1528, 1994.
48. Prechtl JC, Powley TL: B-afferents: A fundamental division of the nervous system mediating homeostasis? Behav Brain Sci 13:289–331, 1990.
49. Ramsey RH: The anatomy of the ligamenta flava. Clin Orthop 44:129–140, 1966.
50. Rhalmi S, Yahia L'H, Newman N, Isler M: Immunohistochemical study of nerves in lumbar spinae ligaments. Spine 18:264–267, 1993.
51. Roaf R: A study of the mechanics of spinal injuries. J Bone Joint Surg 42B:810–823, 1960.
52. Schaible H-G, Grubb BD: Afferent and spinal mechanisms of joint pain. Pain 55:5–54, 1993.
53. Schwarzer AC, Aprill CN, Bogduk N: The sacroiliac joint in chronic low back pain. Spine 20:31–37, 1995.
54. Simonian PT, Routt MLC, Harrington RM, et al: Biomechanical simulation of the anteroposterior compression injury of the pelvis. Clin Orthop 309:245–256, 1994.
55. Snijders CJ, Vleeming A, Stoeckart R: Transfer of lumbosacral load to iliac bones and legs. Part I: Biomechanics of self-bracing of the sacroiliac joints and its significance for treatment and exercise. Clin Biomech 8:285–294, 1993.
56. Stilwell DL: The nerve supply of the vertebral column and its associated structures in the monkey. Anat Rec 125:139–169, 1956.
57. Uhthoff HK: Prenatal development of the ilolumbar ligament. J Bone Joint Surg 75B:93–95, 1993.
58. Vleeming A, Pool-Goudzwaard AL, Stoeckart R, et al: The posterior layer of the thoracolumbar fascia: Its function in load transfer from spine to legs. Spine 20:753–758, 1995.
59. Vleeming A, Stoeckart R, Snijders CJ: The sacrotuberous ligament: A conceptual approach to its dynamic role in stabilizing the sacroiliac joint. Clin Biomech 4:201–203, 1989.
60. Vleeming A, Stoeckart R, Snijders CJ: General introduction (to the sacroiliac joint). In Vleeming A, Mooney V, Snijders C, Dorman T (eds): Low Back Pain and Its Relation to the Sacroiliac Joint. Rotterdam, First Interdisciplinary World Congress on Low Back Pain, 1993, pp 3–63.
61. Vleeming A, Van Wingerdan JP, Snijders CJ, et al: Load application to the sacrotuberous ligament; influences on sacroiliac joint mechanics. Clin Biomech 4:204–209, 1989.
62. Weidenbaum M, Farcyu J-P: Pain syndromes of the lumbar spine. In Floman Y (ed): Disorders of the Lumbar Spine. Rockville, MD, Aspen, 1990.
63. Weinstein JN: The role of neurogenic and non-neurogenic mediators as they relate to pain and the development of osteoarthritis. Spine 105:S356–S361, 1992.
64. White AA, Panjabi MM: Kinematics of the spine. In White AA, Panjabi MM (eds): Clinical Biomechanics of the Spine. Philadelphia, JB Lippincott, 1990, pp 86–125.
65. Williams PL, Warwick R, Dyson M, Bannister LH: Gray's Anatomy. 37th ed. Edinburgh, Churchill Livingstone, 1989.
66. Yahia L-H, Garzon S, Strykowski H, Rivard C-H: Ultrastructure of the human interspinous ligament and ligamentum flavum: A preliminary study. Spine 15:262–268, 1990.
67. Yamamoto I, Panjabi MM, Oxland TR, Crisco JJ: The role of the iliolumbar ligament in the lumbosacral junction. Spine 15:1138–1141, 1990.
68. Yamashita T, Cavanaugh JM, El-Bohy AA, et al: Mechanosensitive afferent units in the lumbar facet joint. J Bone Joint Surg 72A:865–870, 1990.

STEPHEN M. LEVIN, MD

THE IMPORTANCE OF SOFT TISSUES FOR STRUCTURAL SUPPORT OF THE BODY

From the Potomac Back Center
Vienna, Virginia

Reprint requests to:
Stephen M. Levin, MD
Director
Potomac Back Center
1577 Springhill Road
Vienna, VA 22182

Most of us view the skeleton as the frame upon which the soft tissues are draped. The post-and-beam construction of a skyscraper is the favored model for the spine[11] and is used for all biologic structures—the upright spine is regarded as the highest biomechanical achievement. The soft tissues are regarded as stabilizing "guy wires," similar to the curtain walls of steel-framed buildings (Fig. 1).

Skyscrapers are immobile, rigidly hinged, high-energy–consuming, vertically oriented structures that depend on gravity to hold them together. The mechanical properties are Newtonian, Hookian, and linear.[4,5] A skyscraper's flagpole or any weight that cantilevers off the building creates a bending moment in the column that produces instability. The building must be rigid to withstand even the weight of a flag blowing in the wind. The heavier or farther out the cantilever, the stronger and more rigid the column must be (Fig. 2). A rigid column requires a heavy base to support the incumbent load. The weight of the structure produces internal shear forces that are destabilizing and require energy just to keep the structure intact (Fig. 3).

Biologic structures are mobile, flexibly hinged, low-energy–consuming, omnidirectional structures that can function in a gravity-free environment. The mechanical properties are non-Newtonian, nonHookian, and nonlinear.[5] If a human skeletal system functions as a lever, reaching out a hand or casting a fly at the end of a rod is impossible. The calculated forces with such acts break bone, rip muscle, and deplete energy (Fig. 4).

SPINE: State of the Art Reviews—Vol. 9, No. 2, May 1995
Philadelphia, Hanley & Belfus, Inc.

357

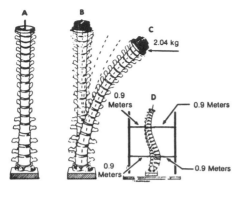

FIGURE 1 (Left). Adult thoracolumbar ligamentous spine, fixed at the base and free at top, under vertical loading, and restrained at midthoracic and midlumbar levels in the anteroposterior plane. *A*, before loading. *B*, during loading. *C*, stability failure occurring under a load of 2.04 kg. *D*, lateral view showing anteroposterior restraints. (From Morris JM, Markolk KL: Biomechanics of the lumbar spine. In American Academy of Orthopaedic Surgeons: Atlas of Orthotics: Biomechanical Principles and Application. St. Louis, Mosby, 1975; with permission.)

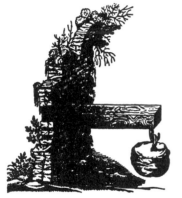

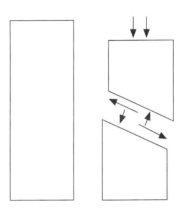

FIGURE 2 (Above, Left). Bending stresses in a beam. (From Galileo: Discorci e dimonstrazioni matematiche intorno a due nuove scienze. Leiden, 1638.)

FIGURE 3 (Above, right). When simple compressive load is applied, both compressive and shear stresses must exist on planes that are oriented obliquely to the line of application to the load.

A post-and-beam cannot be used to model the neck of a flamingo, the tail of a monkey, the wing of a bat, or the spine of a snake (Fig. 5). Because invertebrates do not have bones, there is no satisfactory model to adequately explain the structural integrity of a worm. Post-and-beam modeling in biologic structures could only apply in a perfectly balanced, rigidly hinged, upright spine (Fig. 6). Mobility is out of the equation. The forces needed to keep a column whose center of gravity is constantly changing and whose base is rapidly moving horizontally are overwhelming to contemplate. If we add that the column is composed of many rigid bodies that are hinged together by flexible, almost frictionless joints, the forces are incalculable.[2] The complex cantilevered beams of horizontal spines of quadrupeds and cervical spines in any vertebrate require tall, rigid masts for support[2] that are not usually available.

Since post-and-beam construction has limited use in biologic modeling, other structural models must be explored to determine if a more widely applicable construct can be found. Thompson[14] and, later, Gordon[4] use a truss system similar to those used in bridges for modeling the quadruped spine. Trusses have clear advantages over the post-and-lintel construction of skyscrapers as a structural support system for biologic tissue. Trusses have flexible, even frictionless hinges with no

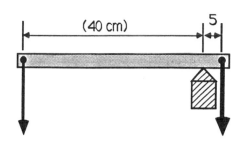

FIGURE 4. A log of 200 kg located 40 cm from the fulcrum requires a muscle reaction force of $8 \times 200 =$ kg. The erectores spinae group can generate a force of about 200–400 kg, which is only a quarter to half of the force that is necessary. Therefore, muscle power alone cannot lift such a load, and another supporting member is required. (Courtesy of Serge Gracovetsky, PhD.)

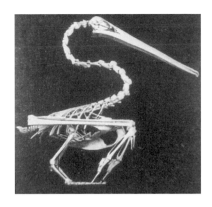

FIGURE 5. Bird skeleton. (Courtesy of California Academy of Sciences, San Francisco.)

bending moments about the joint. The support elements are either in tension or compression only. Loads applied at any point are distributed about the truss as tension or compression (Fig. 7). In post-and-beam construction, the load is locally loaded and creates leverage. There are no levers in a truss, and the load is distributed throughout the structure. A truss is fully triangulated, inherently stable, and cannot be bent without producing large deformations of individual members. Since only trusses are in-

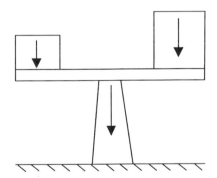

FIGURE 6 *(Left).* Balancing compressive loads.

FIGURE 7 *(Right).* Loading a square and a triangular (truss) frame.

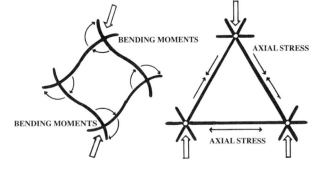

BENDING MOMENTS

AXIAL STRESS

BENDING MOMENTS

AXIAL STRESS

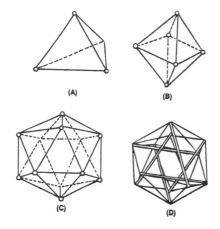

FIGURE 8. *A*, tetrahedron, *B*, octahedron, *C*, icosahedron, and *D*, tension-vectored icosahedron with compression elements within the tension shell.

herently stable with freely moving hinges, it follows that any stable structure with freely moving hinges must be a truss. Vertebrates with flexible joints must therefore be constructed as trusses.

When the tension elements of a truss are wires or ropes, the truss usually becomes unidirectional (see Fig. 7); the element that is under tension will be under compression when turned topsy-turvy. The tension elements of the body (the soft tissues—fascia, muscles, ligaments, and connective tissue) have largely been ignored as construction members of the body frame and have been viewed only as the motors. In loading a truss the elements that are in tension can be replaced by flexible materials such as ropes, wires, or in biologic systems, ligaments, muscles, and fascia. Therefore, the tension elements are an integral part of the construction and not just a secondary support. However, ropes and soft tissue can only function as tension elements, and most trusses constructed with tension members will only function when oriented in one direction. They could not function as mobile, omnidirectional structures necessary for biologic functions. There is a class of trusses called *tensegrity*[3] structures that are omnidirectional so that the tension elements always function in tension regardless of the direction of applied force. A wire bicycle wheel is a familiar example of a tensegrity structure. The compression elements in tensegrity structures "float" in a tension network just as the hub of a wire wheel is suspended in a tension network of spokes.

To conceive of an evolutionary system construction of tensegrity trusses that can be used to model biologic organisms, we must find a tensegrity truss that can be linked in a hierarchical construction. It must start at the smallest subcellular component and

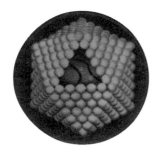

FIGURE 9.   The icosahedral structure of a virus.

must have the potential, like the beehive, to build itself. The structure would be an integrated tensegrity truss that evolved from infinitely smaller trusses that could be, like the beehive cell, both structurally independent and interdependent at the same time. This repetition of forms, like in a hologram, helps in visualizing the evolutionary progression of complex forms from simple ones. This holographic concept seems to apply to the truss model as well.

Architect Buckminster Fuller[3] and sculptor Kenneth Snelson[13] described the truss that fits these requirements, the tensegrity icosahedron. In this structure, the outer shell is under tension, and the vertices are held apart by internal compression "struts" that seem to float in the tension network (Fig. 8).

The tensegrity icosahedron is a naturally occurring, fully triangulated, three-dimensional truss. It is an omnidirectional, gravity-independent, flexibly hinged structure whose mechanical behavior is nonlinear, nonNewtonian, and nonHookian. Independently, Fuller and Snelson use this truss to build complex structures. Fuller's familiar geodesic dome is an example, and Snelson[12] has used it for artistic sculptures that can be seen around the world. Ingber[7,16] and colleagues use the icosahedron for modeling cell construction. Research is underway to use this structure in more complex tissue modeling.[16] Naturally occurring examples that have already been recognized as icosahedra are the self-generating fullerenes (carbon$_{60}$ organic molecules),[8] viruses,[17] clethrins,[1] cells,[15] radiolaria,[6] pollen grains, dandelion balls, blowfish, and several other biologic structures[9] (Fig. 9).

Icosahedra are stable even with frictionless hinges and, at the same time, can easily be altered in shape or stiffness merely by shortening or lengthening one or several tension elements. Icosahedra can be linked in an infinite variety of sizes or shapes in a modular or hierarchical pattern with the tension elements (the muscles, ligaments, and fascia) forming a continuous interconnecting network and with the compression elements (the bones) suspended within that network (Fig. 10). The structure would always maintain the characteristics of a single icosahedron. A shaft, such as a spine, may be built that is omnidirectional and can function equally well in

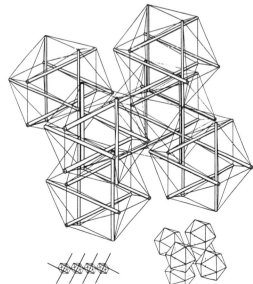

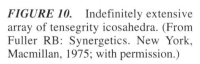

FIGURE 10. Indefinitely extensive array of tensegrity icosahedra. (From Fuller RB: Synergetics. New York, Macmillan, 1975; with permission.)

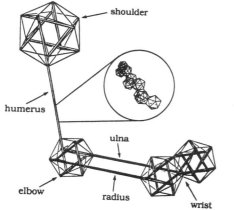

FIGURE 11.   Icosa arm.

tension or compression with the internal stresses always distributed in tension or compression. Because there are no bending moments within a tensegrity structure, they have the lowest energy costs.

Viewed as a model for the spine of humans or any vertebrate species, the tension icosahedron space truss (Fig. 11) with the bones acting as the compressive elements and the soft tissues as the tension elements will be stable in any position, even with multiple joints. They can be vertical or horizontal and assume any posture from ramrod straight to a sigmoid curve (Fig. 12). Shortening one soft tissue element has a rippling effect throughout the structure. Movement is created and a new, instantly stable shape is achieved. It is highly mobile, omnidirectional, and consumes low energy. Tension icosahedrons are unique structures whose constructs, when used as a biologic model, would conform to the natural laws of least energy, laws of mechanics, and the distinct characteristics of biologic tissues. The icosahedron space

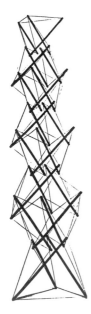

FIGURE 12.   E-C column. (Courtesy of Kenneth Snelson.)

truss is present in biologic structures at the cellular, subcellular, and multicellular levels. Recent research on the molecular structures of organisms such as viruses, subcellular organelles, and whole organisms has shown them to be icosahedra. The very building block of bone, hydroxyapetite, is an icosahedron. In the spine, each subsystem (vertebrae, disks, soft tissues) would be subsystems of the spine metasystem. Each would function as an icosahedron independently and as part of the larger system, as in the beehive analogy.

The icosahedron space truss spine model is a universal, modular, hierarchical system that has the widest application with the least energy cost. As the simplest and least energy-consuming system, it becomes the metasystem to which all other systems and subsystems must be judged and, if they are not simpler, more adaptable, and less energy consuming, rejected. Since this system always works with the least energy requirements, there would be no benefit to nature for spines to function sometimes as a post, sometimes as a beam, sometimes as a truss, or to function differently for different species, conforming to the minimal inventory-maximum diversity concept of Pearce[10] and evolutionary theory.

The icosahedron space truss model could be extended to incorporate other anatomic and physiologic systems. For example, as a "pump" the icosahedron functions remarkably like cardiac and respiratory models, and, so, may be an even more fundamental metasystem for biologic modeling. As suggested by Kroto,[8] the icosahedron template is "mysterious, ubiquitous, and all powerful."

REFERENCES

1. de Duve C: A Guided Tour of the Living Cell. Vol 1. New York, Scientific American Books, 1984.
2. Fielding WJ, Burstein AH, Frankel VH: The nuchal ligament. Spine 1:3–14, 1976.
3. Fuller RB: Synergetics. New York, Macmillan, 1975.
4. Gordon JE: Structures or Why Things Don't Fall Down. New York De Capa Press, 1978.
5. Gordon JE: The Science of Structures and Materials. New York, Scientific American Library, 1988.
6. Haeckel E: Report on the scientific results of the voyage of the H.M.S. Challenger. Vol 18, pt XL. Radiolaria. Edinburgh, 1887.
7. Ingber DE, Jamieson J: Cells as tensegrity structures. Architectural regulation of histodifferentiation by physical forces transduced over basement membrane. In Andersonn LL, Gahmberg CG, Kblom PE (eds): Gene Expression During Normal and Malignant Differentiation. New York, Academic Press, 1985, pp 13–30.
8. Kroto H: Space, stars, C_{60}, and soot. Science 242:1139–1145, 1988.
9. Levin SM: The icosahedron as the three-dimensional finite element in biomechanical support. Proceedings of the Society of General Systems Research Symposium on Mental Images, Values and Reality, Philadelphia, 1986. St. Louis, Society of General Systems Research, 1986, pp G14–G26.
10. Pearce PL: Structure in Nature as a Strategy for Design. Cambridge, MA, MIT Press, 1978.
11. Schultz AB: Biomechanics of the spine. In Nelson L (ed): Low Back Pain and Industrial and Social Disablement. London, American Back Pain Association, 1983, pp 20–25.
12. Schultz DG, Fox HN: Kenneth Snelson, Albright-Knox Art Gallery (catalogue). Buffalo, 1981.
13. Snelson KD: Continuous tension, discontinuous compression structures. U.S. Patent 3,169,611, Washington, DC, U.S. Patent Office, 1965.
14. Thompson D: On Growth and Form. Cambridge, Cambridge University Press, 1961.
15. Wang N, Butler JP, Ingber DE: Microtransduction across the cell surface and through the cytoskeleton. Science 260:1124–1127, 1993.
16. Wendling S: Personal communication. Laboratory of Physical Mechanics, Faculty of Science and Technology, Paris.
17. Wildy P, Home RW: Structure of animal virus particles. Prog Med Virol 5:1–42, 1963.

THOMAS A. DORMAN, MD

ELASTIC ENERGY IN THE PELVIS

Private Practice
San Luis Obispo, California

Portions of this chapter have been excerpted from Dorman TA: Storage and release of elastic energy in the pelvis: Dysfunction, diagnosis and treatment. J Orthop Med 14:54–62, 1992; and Dorman TA, Buchmiller JC, Cohen RE, et al: Energy efficiency during human walking. J Orthop Med 15:64–66, 1993; with permission.

Fish and snakes advance by waves of lateral contraction and relaxation of groups of muscles within metamers. Reptiles with four legs maintain this mode of locomotion. Their body weight is supported directly on the ground. Quadruped walking of mammals is more complex. The body is no longer on the ground, and the organism alternately supports body quadrants over the swing leg so that a quantum increase in coordination and balance is necessary. The complexity of the nervous system and size of the brain parallel the increased intricacy of locomotion and coordination.

Although passive-dynamic walking calls for little action from the nervous system,[36] biped walking represents another increment in complexity. The static support of any structure on legs calls for at least three points of support, a possibility in the quadruped stance. Biped locomotion, on the other hand, is predicated on balance and coordination with continuous movement. Perhaps this is the reason for the additional increase in size of the human brain.[44]

Since Charles Darwin's[16] proposal of a common ancestral origin for *Homo sapiens* and humanoids, it has been assumed that the human biped posture is an evolutionary development from a more primitive quadruped one. The absence of a confirmatory paleontologic link after 150 years of research should raise the consideration that bipedal locomotion and the upright stance represent an earlier, or intrinsic, characteristic of *Homo sapiens*.[9,10,25] The suggestion that mechanical and gravitational influences have contributed to morphologic ontogeny and, by implication, to phylogeny is neither new[8,46] nor passè.[11] In this context it might be interesting to

SPINE: State of the Art Reviews—Vol. 9, No. 2, May 1995
Philadelphia, Hanley & Belfus, Inc.

365

consider the anatomy, comparative anatomy, and physiology of walking in the human frame as not necessarily closely analogous to quadruped walking. This hypothesis should be judged for its usefulness by its outcome; to a clinician, outcome is measured in therapeutics.

THE PHYSIOLOGY OF WALKING

Only a moderate amount of research has been conducted on the dynamic mechanics of walking. Dynamic similarity has been demonstrated, based on the geometry and physics of terrestrial conditions, for quadrupedal mammals.[7] The periodicity was defined in the Froude number, which might serve with some modifications in the analysis of human walking. Studies on the efficiency of locomotion have barely touched on human ambulation[48] but have recorded a paradox.[5] Oxygen consumption in human running is substantially less than calculated from the work done. (Various forms of terrestrial locomotion have similar energy economics[13]). Although a large bibliography has accumulated on gait, the "research front"[49] has been on instrumentation based on EMG and the use of dynamic imaging modalities for comparison of normal and abnormal gait in various conditions. Just as there has been a paucity of interest in the anatomy of the pelvic ring in general and the sacrum in particular, so has there been a deficiency in analysis of the role of these structures in locomotion.[24] There has been a suggestion recently that the anatomy of the human pelvis has evolved, teleologically speaking, to accommodate efficient walking rather than parturition.[1,2,42] This chapter will review the available research from an orthopedic medical perspective. The focus will be on the human pelvis and the sacroiliac articulations.

It is advantageous teleologically for the bipedal organism to conserve energy during locomotion. Conservation can take several forms.

Walking: A Pendulum

A pendulum conserves energy. The kinetic energy is stored in the upswing, as gravitational energy, to be released after the pendulum momentarily stops at the inertia point. A small amount of energy is imparted to the pendulum with each swing—the additional push being just sufficient to compensate for the loss by friction. By this means, the pendulum of a grandfather clock reuses the swing energy time and again, kinetic and gravitational energy alternating, recycling. On observing a walking man, the analogy acquires flesh[4] (which contrasts with the relative inefficiency of quadruped walking[3]). The efficiency of stride length and speed of walking have been evaluated through the study of oxygen consumption.[28] There is an optimal speed of walking for each individual, which can be predicted by physical measurements.[26] These observations support the analogy with a pendulum. Walking begins as a controlled fall. Then, as the pelvis hitches up on the stance leg and the swing leg departs from the ground, the leg gains momentum at first and decelerates before heel contact. The first acceleration occurs from the controlled forward fall, and the deceleration occurs at the end of the swing. Was the decelerating energy dissipated as heat? Some studies have shown that, at least in human running, there is some storage or reuse of energy.[4] The kinetic energy of the decelerating leg apparently is transferred in part into forward locomotion (Newton's Third Law of Physics says that every force is opposed by an equal and opposite force). The upper end of the swing leg, being attached to the pelvis and thence to the trunk, transmits forward locomotion to the body with deceleration. This can be observed in gait-analysis studies, which show uneven acceleration of the trunk during forward progression.

The body wobbles backward and forward during forward walking. To appreciate this wobble, which is superimposed on the overall advancement, it is advantageous to subtract the average forward movement. The wobble of a person walking on a treadmill is thought to represent the cyclic intake and dissipation of kinetic energy in synchrony with the pendular movement of the legs.

Walking is more efficient than running,[12,41] but knowledge of the exact degree of this efficiency is elusive.

Trunk Bobbing

During normal walking, the head (and body) move up and down in the equivalent of a sinusoid wave. What is the fate of the gravitational energy dissipated on the downslope? It is proposed that this energy is largely not converted to heat and lost but is stored in the "walking machine." Part of it is transmitted to forward locomotion, a fall off the stance leg. Part is transmitted into elastic tissues such as the collagen of the ligaments reinforcing the anterior aspect of the hip joint. In long strides just before the rear leg is converted from a stance to a swing leg, tension can be sensed in the front of the hip. This stretch—elastic energy—is promptly released again as the stance leg begins to swing. In fact, it contributes to the acceleration of the swing leg together with the gravitational contribution mentioned earlier.

It is more efficient to carry a weight on the head than in a back pack;[35] the weight on the head presumably does not interfere with the vertical "clockwork mechanism" under discussion here.

ELASTIC ENERGY

The storage of elastic energy has been recognized and taken for granted by the keepers of physiologic knowledge since the turn of the century. Examples include the following.

Respiration, Joint Capsules, and Fasciae

Inspiration is the result of active contraction of intercostal muscles and the diaphragm; the chest expands. The initial phase of expiration is passive, the elastic chest wall collapsing to a smaller volume. Forced expiration calls for muscle action contracting the chest to a smaller volume. The neutral position is known to represent a dynamic neutrality because the lungs collapse to an even smaller volume. The vacuum in the pleural space (sometimes erroneously called negative pressure) stops them from collapse. Therefore, the neutral position of the chest in the intact organism represents a greater degree of pulmonary expansion than would be spontaneous for the lungs alone. In contrast, the chest wall itself is pulled inward somewhat by the elasticity of the lungs proper so its resting posture is more contracted than would be the case without the inward pull of the lungs. The balance, therefore, is one of a dynamic equilibrium. In this instance, the elasticity of the rib cage is balanced by the elasticity of the lungs. The breathing organism needs only shift the balance to and fro a little for the bellows to work. Although the pendulum analogy applies, a better analogy is that of the coiled balance spring of a watch escapement. As discussed in the second chapter, it was during the 1600s when elastic energy was first stored in a spring rather than a gravity pendulum.

As understanding of the walking machine advances, another analogy from the clockmakers' trade applies. Where else in the body is elastic energy stored in each step? It would be advantageous teleologically for the walking machine to use the spring-storage model as extensively as possible. The following discussion will be based mostly on hypothesis because there have been only a few recorded instances of stored elastic energy.

The storage of elastic energy in the ventral ligaments of the interdigital joint capsule can be confirmed by stretching a finger backward and releasing it. From watching the cycle of walking, it seems that elastic energy is stored in the anterior part of the hip capsule (not only by extension but also by internal rotation of the femur). Alignment of the main collagenous fibers in the anterior portion of the hip joint is notable; the fibers are stretched by this movement. This applies to the posterior ligaments of the knee, the so-called ligament of Valois; in the foot, the plantar aponeurosis and the ligaments of the deep arches of the foot are all stretched at the end of the stance phase and all release energy as the limb begins its swing.

The term *fasciae* is used in this chapter to describe the sheets of connective tissue made up predominantly of woven collagen fibers, which were once referred to as surgical fasciae and intermuscular septae. Ligaments are connective tissue structures that bind bone to bone. Tendons are connective tissue structures that bind muscle to bone and, occasionally, muscle to muscle. Fasciae are flat sheets of collagenous material that bind other elements of the musculoskeletal system to each other and traverse the body widely.[34] The aphorism that *the fascia is continuous* is worth repeating.

Storage of Elastic Energy

A ballerina in the fifth position winds up her legs each in external rotation, so tension is created between them. Each is wound up in an opposite direction on the pelvis. When the ballerina initiates the pirouette with a slight muscle-induced knee extension, the stored energy is released and converted to a vertical jump. In dancing circles this force has been recognized since before the days of Diaghalev. In this example, where is the elastic energy stored? Some is stored in the foot (as in the case of the posterior stance leg discussed earlier), some in the medial collateral ligaments of the knee, and some in the anterior ligaments of the hip joint. But anyone who assumes this position will sense the tension in the enveloping fasciae of calf and thigh. A crouched runner in a start position similarly stores energy in his calf, although much of this elasticity is stored in the triceps surae. Hitherto, conventional wisdom has ascribed the functions of wrapping and compartmentalization to fascia. It is proposed here that fascia has the additional function of the *storage of elastic energy*. The instances where this has been proved through research or accepted by convention are not many,[50] but perhaps this discussion might serve as a springboard for new research.

THE LOCUS OF ENERGY STORAGE

Since the early research on locomotion,[14,47] it has been assumed that the storage of elastic energy has been imputed to the *muscles*; even recent authoritative researchers have accepted a role in elastic storage merely to the tendons of muscles.[6] It seems, however, that this ascription has been arbitrary. The contractile elements of muscles—the actin and myosin—are not inherently elastic; the storage is therefore much more suitably ascribed to collagen and elastin, i.e., the fascial component of the *myofascial* structures and to ligaments proper.

In the case of the spring ligament of the foot, it is easy to understand how the talus is supported by elastic tension between calcaneum and navicular. The weight of the body transmitted via the talus stretches the spring ligament, which releases its energy to the uprising foot. In final analysis, it can be reasonably assumed that the energy is stored in electrostatic forces in the outer electron shells of the stretched atoms, making up the collagen molecules and strands, right inside the spring ligaments.[38]

On the other hand is the example of a discus thrower who has wound up his torso just before starting the swing that will eventually transmit all his elastic, muscular, and kinetic energy into the flying discus. Can an analysis be made of the *exact locus* of the stored elastic energy at that moment? In the case of the coiled watch spring in the mechanical wrist watch escapement, can we analyze where *in the spring* the elastic energy is stored? In both cases the answer has to be that the energy is stored *diffusely* in the whole structure. (The storage of a small amount of energy in the spring cannot be ascribed to a group of molecules at one end of it, and it is proposed here that this analogy can be applied to a certain extent to the body's fascia.) Just as the fascia is anatomically continuous, so it is with the stored energy. The storage is diffuse.

THE RESEARCH FRONT

Over the past half century, Anglo-American research has insisted on measurements. This *reductionist* approach has yielded much excellent information. By nature, however, certain subjects lend themselves better to a *systems analysis*.[20,22,23] Therefore, studies on the use of energy in the whole organism are most likely to provide answers on the function of the diffuse dynamic organ system of the fascia and ligaments as a whole. It might be that walking bipeds store energy in the fascia of the whole body and release it with each step. Perhaps connective tissue could be viewed as an *organ for energy storage* just as dermatologists have changed the concept of the skin from integument to organ.

Torque

With walking, the arms swing alternately and synchronously. In fact, the upper girdle rotates back and forth with each step. The angular momentum and acceleration are proportionate to the speed of walking. An horological analogy is available. The store of energy in a horizontal circular so-called pendulum, which is really a flywheel torqued on a suspensory spring, was invented in the Black Forest in 1881 and serves as the basis for the famous 400-day clock. Though not suspended, the upper girdle functions the same way. Torque is stored in the spine (and a little gravitational energy in the rising and falling arms). With the arms bound or the upper girdle restrained with a haversack frame, walking is fatiguing, chaffing, and inefficient, as confirmed by measurements of oxygen consumption when the torso is in a brace.[27] The pelvic girdle swivels with each step in time with the swing leg and in alternating synchrony with the upper girdle. Is there room to suppose that elastic energy is stored in the pelvic girdle itself?

The Spinal Engine

Gracovetsky[24] has explained the mechanisms by which the small muscles of the spine convert their contractions into locomotion. Side bending is converted to torque through the "gear box" of the zygoapophyseal joints. Finally, pelvic rotation activates the legs.

Immobilization of the trunk retards the efficiency of walking,[43] as judged by oxygen use. Does this represent an interference with the action of the spinal muscles in the "spinal engine," or does it mean that there is interference with the storage and release of elastic energy (torque), which might enhance the pendular (flywheel) efficiency of the "walking machine"?

PELVIC DYNAMICS

The old idea that the three pelvic bones are immobile serves as a reminder that widely held views are not always correct.[51,52] The relative movement of the ilia versus the sacrum and each other in space, in time, and with the activity of walking in health and disease are under study, and a number of relative movements, axes of rotation, and other dynamics have been suggested. The research available so far points to variation and differences.[21] The presence of movement and the presence of asymmetry are emerging as the norm. All of these measurements are based on anatomic observations of the bony parts. The problem is confounded by the complexity of bony geometry, the extraordinary degree of variation, and the extreme difficulty in defining a reference point. Are the wrong questions being asked? Perhaps it would be better to ask questions about the storage capacity of the elastic structures and about hysteresis. In contemporary podiatry, the role of ligaments in the storage of elastic energy with stepping is gaining acceptance (see chapter 8). However, it can be stated with confidence that the iliac bones move versus each other and the sacrum with each step. Asymmetry of the inclination of the pelvis is common. It is enhanced in dysfunction and painful conditions and restored toward symmetry with effective healing, whether manual or other.[31]

The relationship of torque at the sacrum to weightbearing with the alternation of stepping in walking has been demonstrated recently[45] and probably represents the first step in understanding the connection between the passive dynamic walking model of McGeer[36] and the synchronous flywheel (or rotary pendulum) of the upper trunk, shoulders and arms, sprung on the elastic spine.

Looking at ligaments and fasciae only from the perspective of the storage of energy, one might ask where the ligaments are most plentiful. Here, the pelvis comes into its own. The posterior sacroiliac ligaments are by far the heftiest ligaments in the body. It has been recognized that the sacrum is *suspended* from the ilia and, hence, the whole weight of the organism is suspended by these ligaments. The strength was attributed to this function. However, the function may be that of an hierarchical icasahedron, functioning as a whole, so that the local concentration of ligament tissue may not necessarily have a role in suspension after all.[32,33] Now that it is recognized that torque occurs through the sacroiliac joints with each step, perhaps these massive posterior sacroiliac ligaments should be regarded as analogous to the mainspring of a clock. There is no reason why a short but strong spring should not store a great deal of energy in a small moment. Of course, only a very small amount of movement can occur at the sacroiliac joints.

Sacroiliac joints serve as a bracing mechanism or as shock absorbers in jumping and falling,[5] but it is likely that this is also part of their role in each step. What, then, is the movement at the sacroiliac joints with stepping, where exactly is the energy stored, and when in the cycle of gait? Recent evidence suggests that walking normally is more efficient than the sum of the parts. The implication is that energy is stored antigravitationally and through elasticity in the soft tissues.

TWO EXPERIMENTS

Previous experience with injuries of the soft tissues has promoted interest in their physiologic effects.[14,34,41] The two studies described below explored energy efficiency during walking. Both were performed within the framework of student senior projects at California Polytechnic University in San Luis Obispo, California. The first study was carried out in 1992, the second in 1994.

The Efficiency of Walking

The first experiment tested the hypothesis that the soft tissues of the body (fascia and ligaments), through their elastic properties and swinging of the limbs, enhance the efficiency of human walking. The presumed effects are through the mechanisms of storage and release of elastic and kinetic pendular energy.[19]

Eleven healthy volunteers between the ages of 19 and 24 were selected for the study. Table 1 summarizes the personal data; the volunteers fasted for 4 hours prior to testing.

For the purpose of the experiment, the composite function of walking was divided into components: (1) the rise and fall of the body with each step (head rise), (2) arm swing, calculated twice, (3) leg swing, calculated twice, (4) shoulder swing, and (5) basal rate of oxygen consumption. The components of walking were measured to test a portion of the hypothesis that predicted that the body is more efficient when it is able to function as a whole.

Angular rotation of the shoulders, length of the stride, height of head rise, and range of arm swing were measured using mechanical and optical devices during unrestricted walking. Angular rotation of the upper trunk was calculated from the rotation of the shoulders. This was recorded in each person by placing a wire extension across one shoulder. Shoulder movement, together with the remaining components, was recorded on a paper backdrop by an observer from a single observation point. The speed of the walking cycle (rhythm) was recorded with a metronome. Each walking component was performed separately, maintaining range of movement and periodicity as recorded from that person's unrestricted walking.

To determine the effects of upper body movement on energy consumption during walking, a body jacket was used to immobilize the spine. The immobilization provided a comparison between restricted and unrestricted walking. The adjustable body jacket was constructed by a prosthetist/orthotist and designed to fit one of the subjects whose build was average. It was bivalved with three lateral Velcro closures made of $\frac{1}{8}$-inch Kydex and lined with plastozote foam. An adjustable head brace restricting neck rotation was attached to the posterior surface of the body jacket. The person's arms were strapped across the front of the chest to restrict arm swing. The jacket restricted all body movement above the pelvis in all the volunteers, and it restricted the pelvic region only slightly.

OXYGEN CONSUMPTION

Human oxygen consumption is a measure of energy expenditure.[28] Oxygen use

TABLE 1. Personal Data of Study Participants

Subject	Age	Walking Speed/MPH	Walking Cycle/Min	Ht/cm	Wt/kg
1M	21	3.4	110	182.0	74.8
2M	20	3.4	107	185.4	74.8
3F	24	3.4	104	167.6	60.8
4M	20	3.6	100	180.3	73.0
5M	22	3.5	99	182.0	76.2
6M	20	3.3	98	175.3	66.8
7M	21	3.4	108	177.8	66.8
8F	20	3.3	102	175.3	61.2
9M	22	3.7	107	188.0	78.5
10M	19	3.6	108	177.8	79.5
11M	21	3.8	107	182.9	74.8

TABLE 2.   Oxygen Consumption for Each Walking Component

Subject	Restricted Walking*	Unrestricted Walking*	Shoulder Swing*	Arm Swing*	Leg Swing*	Head Rise*	Standing Basal*	Sitting Basal*
1M	1.665	1.014	0.037	0.294	0.642	0.348	0.413	0.413
2M	0.940	0.786	0.018	0.020	0.604	0.449	0.310	0.350
3F	1.426	1.325	0.070	0.042	0.820	0.464	0.434	0.274
4M	1.891	1.500	0.212	0.220	0.627	0.642	0.465	0.245
5M	1.134	0.921	0.118	0.457	1.040	0.599	0.354	0.354
6M	1.459	1.273	0.040	0.035	0.735	0.591	0.445	0.445
7M	1.377	1.226	0.053	0.027	0.673	0.337	0.310	0.297
8F	1.051	0.880	0.068	0.304	0.382	0.338	0.260	0.260
9M	1.483	1.238	0.060	0.083	0.633	0.279	0.460	0.476
10M	1.358	1.215	0.120	0.020	0.468	0.536	0.377	0.377
11M	1.203	0.854	0.092	0.256	1.090	0.481	0.337	0.337

* liters O_2 consumed per kg/hr.

was measured with a metabolator, an inverted cylindrical drum that is filled with oxygen and submerged in deionized water. Oxygen is inspired, and exhaled carbon dioxide is removed from the closed system. The residual volume of oxygen is represented graphically by a pen on a rotating drum. Each breath is represented by a rise and fall of the pen, causing a graph to be drawn. The area graphed by the pen was bisected by a line drawn through its center with a ruler, giving the slope and allowing a calculation of the rate of oxygen consumption.

   Three sets of measurements were performed on each volunteer: oxygen consumption during (1) restricted walking, (2) unrestricted walking, and (3) movement of each component of walking. Each measurement was started after the volunteer reached a steady state. All walking was on a level treadmill with variable speed. Basal rates of standing oxygen consumption during rest were recorded for each person. A sitting basal rate of oxygen consumption, recorded for most volunteers, was found to be very close to the standing rate. For five individuals, it was assumed that these basal rates were the same. To calculate the contribution of shoulder rotation while limiting the effect of lower body movement, the volunteer was measured in a sitting position. A single speed of walking was used for each person to ensure consistency. Measurements for restricted walking, at each person's maximum speed, were recorded first since restricted walking was likely to be slower than an individual's natural speed of walking. After the person reached a steady state, recording was repeated until three consistent slopes were obtained. This was followed by unrestricted walking at the same speed. During unrestricted walking, a weight belt weighing the same as the body jacket (2.045 kg) was worn.

RESULTS

   Oxygen consumption for each walking component and for the sum of the parts are listed in Tables 2 and 3, respectively. Table 3 summarizes the differences between the calculated sum of the components of walking and the measurements for unrestricted and for restricted walking. These results were found by the repeated measure t-test to have p value of < 0.005. Calculated standard deviations for the differences are noted. These values were calculated from the slope of the line obtained on the moving drum of the metabolator and represent the O_2 use. Figure 1 illustrates the difference in oxygen consumption between restricted and unrestricted walking for all the subjects. Figure 2 shows the same data as well as a calculation of the O_2 use based on the sum of the components of walking. To determine the oxygen con-

TABLE 3. Oxygen Consumption for the Sum of the Walking Components

Subject	Sum Comp*	DiffR/U%#S D 16.092	DSum/U^ SD 55.029
1M	1.731	64.0	70.7
2M	1.401	19.6	78.2
3F	1.831	7.6	38.2
4M	2.170	26.0	44.4
5M	2.570	23.0	178.0
6M	1.850	14.6	45.0
7M	1.400	12.3	14.2
8F	1.352	19.4	53.6
9M	1.530	19.8	23.7
10M	1.521	11.8	25.2
11M	2.260	40.9	164.0

* liters O_2 consumed per kg/hr.
# Restricted walking versus unrestricted walking: O_2 use in percent.
^ Sum of walking components versus unrestricted walking: O_2 use in percent.

sumption required for each of the individual components, the standing basal O^2 consumption was subtracted from each. The exception was the calculation for shoulder swing. Here the sitting basal rate of O^2 consumption was subtracted (when measured, and the standing basal rate substituted in five subjects, as a close approximation) because the subjects were in a sitting position during the test (to limit pelvic rotation). For testing arm and leg swings, one side was tested and the results doubled. Therefore, the sum of the components included the standing basal, shoulder swing, arm swing, leg swing, and head rise. Figure 3 illustrates the contribution of each component to walking.

DISCUSSION

The findings of this study confirmed the hypothetical role of ligaments in storage and release of elastic energy and the role of the limbs as pendula, outlined ear-

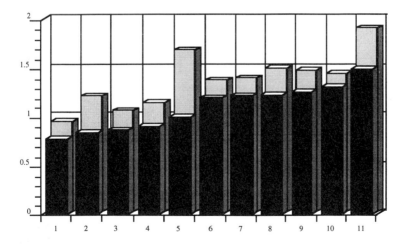

FIGURE 1. Restricted versus unrestricted (front columns) walking in liters of O_2 per kg/hr consumed.

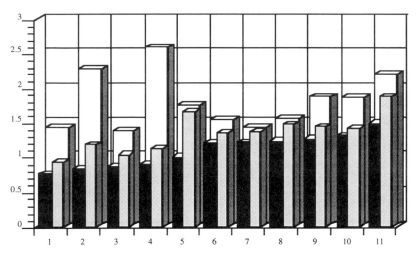

FIGURE 2. All components (back) versus restricted (higher front) and unrestricted (front lower) walking in liters of O_2 per kg/hr consumed.

lier in this chapter, in the case of human walking. Storage of elastic energy historically has been attributed to muscles, their myofascial structures, and tendons.[6,14,34,47] An analysis of the exact locus of energy storage, in the spring of a wristwatch for example, cannot be defined because elasticity is diffused throughout the spring. This consideration applies, it seems, equally to elastic function of ligaments and fascia. In addition to binding elements of the musculoskeletal system together, it has been proposed that fasciae play a role in the transmission of forces within the body.[17,24] It is reasonable to assume that the pendular movements of the legs alternate and transfer the kinetic energy from one side to the other. As the legs alternate their role in stance and swing, and as the sacroiliac joints move with each half stride, the pelvic ligaments act as a spring.

This study showed that pendular leg movements constitute an important component in the energy efficiency of walking. Through consideration of the upper

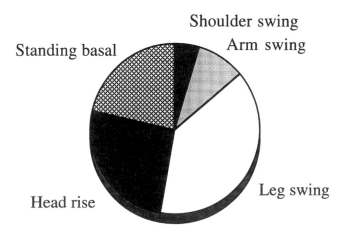

FIGURE 3. The contributions of the components of walking.

body's contribution to the overall efficiency of walking, it was possible to isolate the role of the trunk, neck, and upper limbs with a corset. Increased efficiency was found in the unrestricted condition. A method of restricting the movement of the lower limbs from swinging and allowing walking at the same time could not be found. The implication that elastic and antigravitational pendular energy is stored and released in the pelvis and legs is supported, therefore, only indirectly. For the same reason, the same consideration applies to the rise and fall of the whole body, the "head rise," which was measured but not restricted in a separate walking experiment.

This study hypothesized that elastic and mechanical energy contribute to the efficiency in walking. The difference between the amount of energy used in unrestricted walking and that required for the sum of the components suggests that energy is conserved. Individuals walking while their upper trunk is restricted use more oxygen; that is, they walk with less mechanical efficiency than when unrestricted. This shows that upper trunk movements enhance the efficiency in walking, presumably through the clocklike mechanisms of gravitational and elastic pendulums.

Energy Efficiency Before and After Prolotherapy

The role of ligaments and fascia in the storage of elastic energy has been reviewed above. The second study conducted at California Polytechnic University sought to test the idea that a normally aligned pelvis functions with greater efficiency than one with somatic dysfunction.

The role of prolotherapy in the management of back pain related to sacral dysfunction and ligament insufficiency has been tested clinically.[37,40] Prolotherapy has produced hyperplasia of tissue with an increase in collagen in animal[29] and human tissue,[30] and it has been used to improve the mechanical strength of human knee ligaments.[39] The use of Ongley's technique has made permanent changes in the propensity of patients to experience recurrent pelvic somatic dysfunction.[31] Additionally, patients with back pain who are successfully treated with this technique move with greater ease; and an increase in range of movement occurs.[30] Was it possible that after the abolition of the tendency to somatic dysfunction and an improvement in pelvic ligaments with prolotherapy that the newly discovered function of ligaments—storage and release of elastic energy—was also improved? Is so, would patients walk with greater efficiency after treatment? Would their oxygen consumption decrease for comparable work in walking?

PARTICIPANTS AND TECHNIQUE

Nine patients who were undergoing treatment at the time of the senior project participated in the study. Patients who were undergoing treatment but who were not included those who refused, who lived at a great distance, and two who were so incapacitated at first that they could not walk independently. The demographic data of the patients are summarized in Table 4.

The technique was identical to that used in the first experiment.

MEASUREMENTS

Two sets of measurements were performed on each person: oxygen consumption before treatment and three months after. Each measurement was started after the subject reached a steady state. All walking was on a level treadmill with variable speed. At the initial encounter, the patients were asked to walk at their maximum

TABLE 4. Demographic Data

Pt. ID/Sex	Age	Ht (cm)	Wt (kg)	O_2 (Basal Standing)	O_2 (W1)	O_2(W2)	O_2L/kg/ km(1)*	O_2L/kg/ km(2)*
RB/M	36	168.91	83.5	0.266	0.546		0.256	
MG/M	56	171.45	80.0	0.189	0.505	0.526	0.202	0.158
JH/M	38	177.80	111.3	0.369	0.388	0.490	0.180	0.132
HM/F	68	167.64	90.9	0.220	0.430	0.324	0.380	0.145
SD/F	28	162.56	65.9	0.170	0.432	0.314	0.665	0.243
AF/M	50	172.72	78.2	0.288	0.742	0.763	0.239	0.109
PF/F	31	173.99	64.9	0.286	0.775	0.846	0.127	0.117
SE/F	47	167.64	85.4	0.175	0.601	3.250	0.220	0.200
HD/F	30	160.02	60.9	0.229	1.139	0.729	0.371	0.146

* Oxygen consumed by each subject measured in liters per kilogram of body weight divided by kilometers walked. O_2L/kg/km(1) refers to the patients' original maximum walking speed retested after treatment; O_2L/kg/km(2)* represents their O_2 consumption at their new maximal speed.

speed. At the second encounter—after treatment—the patients were asked to walk at their new maximum speed and at their previous maximum speed. This was achieved by setting the treadmill to the individual's previously recorded speed. After the patient reached a steady state, recording was repeated until two consistent slopes were obtained. Baseline oxygen consumption measurements were obtained repeatedly. Tests were performed 4 hours or more after a meal. Patients' height, weight, pulse, and blood pressures were recorded. Stride length and arm swing during walking were noted. None of the observations varied unexpectedly.

RESULTS

All but one of the patients (R.B.) reported that they were substantially improved symptomatically at the time of the repeat test. The metabolic rate was measured in liters of oxygen consumed per minute. All other data were derived by calculations. Corrections were made for standard temperature and barometric pressure as recorded on the relevant days in order to subtract water vapor pressure in the canister.

Figure 4 summarizes the changes in oxygen consumption before and after treatment per distance walked (work done). The patients (except R.B., who is not graphed) improved symptomatically. They were able to walk faster after treatment. Oxygen consumption at their initial maximal speed failed to show a consistent improvement. However, at their new (and increased) speed, consumption per distance walked (work done) dropped. It was concluded that once a patient's condition improved, the best function was at a higher speed. The average increased efficiency in walking was 38.3%, as calculated from O_2 consumption per distance walked.

These results were found by the repeated measure t-test to have p value of < 0.013 (and df = 7). Calculated standard deviations for the differences are noted.

Patient R.B. reported that his condition improved after the treatment, but subsequently deteriorated with another form of leg pain and before the second measurement. He is believed to have developed a posterolateral displacement of a fragment of the L5–S1 intervertebral disk. He was unable to cooperate fully with the second measurement, and the data indicate a deterioration in his condition.

One of the patients (S.E.) barely improved objectively but did improve symptomatically. About 6 months after treatment, the patient developed cervical spondylopathy necessitating surgical decompression. This was thought to account for the persistence of an inefficient gait.

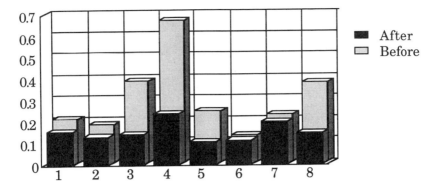

FIGURE 4. Changes in oxygen consumption before and after treatment per distance walked (work done) in liters of O_2 per kg/hr.

DISCUSSION

The contemporary research front in orthopedic medicine implies that soft tissue injuries can be responsible for persistent and recurrent somatic dysfunction. This study focused on the pelvis. In cases of persistent pelvic dysfunction attributed clinically to ligament relaxation, energy efficiency during walking is impaired. After treatment, which includes prolotherapy to the affected ligaments (mainly the posterior sacroiliac ligaments), energy efficiency of walking is improved. This improvement supports the underlying hypothesis.

The subjects were selected carefully by clinical criteria. They were diagnosed as having significant pelvic somatic-dysfunction with ligament relaxation as a cause of their severe and persistent pain. They served as their own controls. With the exception of S.E., no remarkable discrepancies were noted.

Why did the patients exhibit increased efficiency at their faster walking speeds? The synchrony of walking at an individual's optimal speed has been defined in quadruped and biped walking as the Froude number.[5] Presumably when well, restricting the natural speed, from what would be normally brisk walking, is less efficient. This observation was not anticipated when the experiment was planned.

This study's findings support two previously mooted observations: that prolotherapy is effective in the management of select cases of back pain and dysfunction and that ligaments play an important role in the storage and release of elastic energy in walking.

CONCLUSION

This chapter suggests that ligaments and fasciae in the pelvis store elastic energy during walking and that, due to the peculiar arrangement of the sacrum in human anatomy, dysfunction of the pelvic mechanism is often a source of back pain. The clinical diagnosis and practical therapeutics by orthopedic medical means are discussed. Increased efficiency in walking after treatment with prolotherapy is demonstrated, supporting a hypothesis regarding the role of the sacrum and its supporting ligaments in walking.

REFERENCES

1. Abitbol M: Evolution of the ischial spine and the pelvic floor in the hominoidea. Am J Phys Anthropol 75:53–67, 1988.

2. Abitbol M: Evolution of the lumbosacral angle. Am J Phys Anthropol 72:361–372, 1987.
3. Abitbol MM: Effect of posture and locomotion on energy expenditure. Am J Phys Anthropol 77:191–199, 1988.
4. Alexander RM: Biomechanics. London, Chapman & Hall, 1975.
5. Alexander RM: Elastic Mechanisms in Animal Movement. Cambridge, England, Cambridge University Press, 1988.
6. Alexander RM: Energy-saving mechanisms in walking and running. J Exp Biol 160:55–69, 1991.
7. Alexander RM, Jayes AS: A dynamic similarity hypothesis for the gaits of quadrupedal mammals. J Zoology 207A:467–482, 1983.
8. Berg LS: Nomogenesis or Evolution Determined by Law. Cambridge, MA, MIT Press, 1969 (translated from Russian; original, 1922).
9. Berge C, Kasmierczak JB: Effects of size and locomotor adaptations on the hominid pelvis: Evaluation of Australopithecine bipedality with a new multivariate method. Folia Primatol 46:185–204, 1986.
10. Brown F, Harris J, Leakey R, Walker A: Early Homo erectus skeleton from west lake Turkana, Kenya. Nature 316:788–792, 1985.
11. Carter RD: Mechanical loading history and skeletal biology. J Biomech 20:1095–1109, 1987.
12. Cavagna G: Aspects of efficiency and inefficiency of terrestrial locomotion. In Biomechanics VI-A. Baltimore, University Park Press, 1978, pp 3–22.
13. Cavagna GA, Heglund NC, Taylor RC: Mechanical work in terrestrial locomotion: Two basic mechanisms for minimizing energy expenditure. Am J Physiol 233:R243–R261, 1977.
14. Cavagna GA, Saibene FP, Margaria R: Mechanical work in running. J Appl Physiol 19:249–256, 1964.
15. Dananberg HJ: Subtle gait malfunction and chronic musculoskeletal pain. J Orthop Med 14:18–25, 1992.
16. Darwin C: The Descent of Man and Selection in Relation to Sex. 6th ed. 1871.
17. Dorman TA: Storage and release of elastic energy in the pelvis: Dysfunction , diagnosis, and treatment. J Orthop Med 14:54–62, 1992.
18. Dorman TA, Buchmiller JC, Cohen RE, et al: Energy efficiency during human walking. J Orthop Med 15:64–66, 1993.
19. Dorman T, Ravin T: Diagnosis and Injection Techniques in Orthopedic Medicine. Baltimore, Williams & Wilkins, 1991.
20. Elsasser WM: Reflections on a Theory of Organisms. Freligsburgh, Canada, Orbis Publishing, 1987.
21. Fryette HH: Principles of Osteopathic Technic. Colorado Springs, CO, American Academy of Osteopathy, 1954.
22. Fuller RB: Synergetics. New York, Macmillan, 1982.
23. Gleick J: Chaos: Making a New Science. Middlesex, England, Penguin Books, 1987.
24. Gracovetsky S: The Spinal Engine. New York, Springer-Verlag, 1988.
25. Hasegawa M, Kishino H, Yano T: Man's place in hominoidae as inferred from molecular clocks of DNA. J Mol Evol 26:132–147, 1987.
26. Holt KG, Hamill J, Andres RO: Predicting the minimal energy costs of human walking. Med Sci Sports Exerc 23:491–498, 1991.
27. Inman VT: Human locomotion. Can Med Assoc J 94:1047–1057, 1966.
28. Inman VT, Ralston JH, Todd F: Human Walking. Baltimore, Williams & Wilkins, 1981.
29. King Liu Y, Tipton C, Matthews RD, et al: An in situ study of the influence of a sclerosing solution in rabbit medial collateral ligaments and its junction strength. Conn Tiss Res 11:95–102, 1983.
30. Klein R, Dorman T, Johnson C: Prolotherapy in back pain. J Neurol Orthop Med Surg 10:123–126, 1989.
31. LaCourse M, Moore M, Davis V, et al: A report on the asymmetry of iliac inclination: A study comparing normal, laterality and change in a patient population with painful sacro-iliac dysfunction treated with prolotherapy. J Orthop Med 12:3, 1990.
32. Levin SM: The ichosahedron as the three dimensional finite element in biomechanical support. A natural hierarchical system. Presented at the annual meeting of the North American Academy of Manual Medicine, Philadelphia, 1986.
33. Levin SM: Proceedings of the 30th annual meeting of the Society of General Systems Research, Philadelphia 1:G14–26, 1986.
34. Macintosh JE, Bogduk N: Basic biomechanics pertinent to the study of the lumbar disc. J Man Med 5:52–578, 1990.
35. Maloiy GMO, Heglund NC, Prager LM, et al: Energetic costs of carrying loads: Have African women discovered an economic way? Nature 319:668–669.
36. McGeer T: Passive dynamic walking. Int J Robotics Res 9:62–82, 1990.

37. Mooney V, Klein R, Eek CJ, DeLong B: Prolotherapy. J Spine Disord 6:23–33, 1993.
38. Nimni ME: Collagen, Structure and Function. Encyclop Hum Biol 2:559–574, 1991.
39. Ongley MJ, Dorman TA, Eek BC, et al: Ligament instability of knees: A new approach to treatment. Man Med 3:151–154, 1988.
40. Ongley MJ, Klein RG, Dorman TA, et al: A new approach to the treatment of chronic back pain. Lancet 2:143–146, 1987.
41. Pierrynowski M, Winter D, Norman R: Transfers of mechanical energy within the total body and mechanical efficiency during treadmill walking. Ergonomics 23:147–156, 1980.
42. Rak Y: Lucy's pelvic anatomy: Its role in bipedal gait. J Hum Evol 20:283–290, 1991.
43. Ralston HJ: Effects of immobilization of various body segments on the energy cost of human locomotion. Proc 2nd I.E.A. Conf Dortmund 1964. Ergonomics (suppl):53, 1965.
44. Sinclair ARE, Leakey MD: Migration of hominid bipedalism. Nature 324:307–308, 1986.
45. Stevens A: Side bending and axial rotation of the sacrum inside the pelvic girdle. Proceedings of the First International Congress on Low Back Pain and the Sacro-Iliac Joint, San Diego, November 1992.
46. Thompson DW: On growth and form. Cambridge, England. Cambridge University Press, 1961 (original, 1917, 1946).
47. Thys H, Faraggiana T, Margaria R: Utilization of muscle elasticity in exercise. J Apply Physiol 32:491–494, 1972.
48. Tucker VA: The energetic cost of moving about. Am Scientist 63:413–419, 1975.
49. Vaughn K: Biomechanics of human gait: An annotated bibliography. Capetown, South Africa, Department of Biomedical Engineering, University of Capetown, 1982.
50. Vleeming A, Stoeckart R, Snijders CJ: The sacrotuberous ligament: A conceptual approach to its dynamic role in stabilizing the sacro-iliac joint. Clin Biomech 4:201–203, 1989.
51. Weisl H: The movement of the sacro-iliac joint. Acta Anat 23:1955.
52. Weisl H: The relation of movement to structure in the sacro-iliac joint [doctoral thesis]. Manchester, England, University of Manchester, 1953.

STEPHEN M. LEVIN, MD

THE SACRUM IN THREE-DIMENSIONAL SPACE

From the Potomac Back Center
Vienna, Virginia

Reprint requests to:
Stephen M. Levin, MD
Director
Potomac Back Center
1577 Springhill Road
Vienna, VA 22182

Biologic structure must obey all the rules of physics and mechanics.[12] There can be no exceptions. The intricacies of pelvic mechanics should not be a mystery. The laws of physics acting on a body in space are well known, and the methods of applying these laws have been standardized.

A usual approach in biomechanics is to look at the anatomy and try to decipher the role it plays in body stability and movement. An alternative method might be to envision the requirements necessary to perform a function and then try to understand how this is done by the organism. Often, the kinematics (movement without regard to forces) is studied without an understanding of the kinetics (the forces affecting movement). Even less attention is paid to statics (the equilibrium of bodies at rest). Since, first, the body must exist as a structure that is stable and fixed in space, it seems logical to try to understand the statics before exploring the dynamics. The sacrum may be the hub of activity and stability, at least in bipeds, and therefore seems a likely object of investigation. The sacrum appears to be the base of the loadbearing column, the spine. The loadbearing column or wall of a building is the most rigid and rigidly fixed member of that structure. Its base must be on firm footing. The rigidity necessary to bear loads and forces is the antithesis of flexibility needed for movement. What are the forces that stabilize the sacrum, and how can the rigidly stable sacrum move without the body structure collapsing?

A standard engineering tool for determining forces acting on a body that is stable in space is a free-body diagram. A disembodied structure is diagrammed to show the forces acting upon it.

SPINE: State of the Art Reviews—Vol. 9, No. 2, May 1995
Philadelphia, Hanley & Belfus, Inc.

381

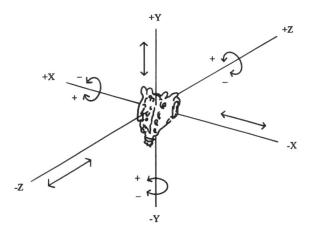

FIGURE 1. The right-handed Cartesian orthogonal coordinate system. The point of intersection of the three axes (here the sacrum) is called the origin. The positive and negative translations and rotations are defined by convention.

Known forces are diagrammed as vectors of force, and the counterbalancing forces that keep the body fixed in space can then be calculated. In a Cartesian coordinate system, a free body can rotate around three axes (x, y, z) and translate in three planes (xy, xz, yz) (Fig. I). White and Punjabi[15] use this concept when describing spinal mechanics, and it is now widely used in the biomechanics literature for describing movement and forces in the musculoskeletal system.[1,16] Convention labels these movement possibilities "six degrees of freedom." However, in biomechanics it seems more logical to describe 12 degrees of freedom, six positive and six negative. A body can be described as rotating positively or negatively around an axis or translating in a plane positively (clockwise) or negatively (counterclockwise).

The interactive forces within the parent structure are usually ignored, for simplicity, so that only the forces of gravity and external applied forces are considered. This works well in buildings and similar structures because what the interactive forces are is usually clear, and they can be readily calculated. In biologic structures the problem is more confusing because the members of the whole organism are

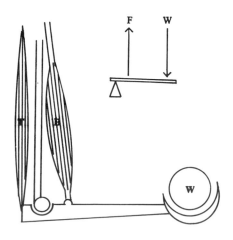

FIGURE 2. Free-body diagram of forces acting on the elbow.

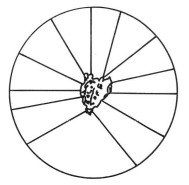

FIGURE 3. The sacrum as the hub of a wire wheel.

highly interactive. For example, a free-body diagram of the forces acting on an elbow joint looks like Figure 2. The force generated by the biceps muscle can be calculated readily. However, the biceps is a two-joint muscle, and as it contracts it creates a moment around the glenohumeral joint that is not part of the free-body diagram. The glenohumeral joint would need to be stabilized to keep the elbow from flying off in space. The triceps muscle would contract to do this (out of the diagram), but this would then put an extensor force on the elbow (back to the diagram). This, in turn, would need to be counterbalanced by the biceps in a feedback loop, throwing off all previous calculations. It would do no good to include the glenohumeral joint in the original free-body diagram because the forces on the scapulothoracic joint would then need to be considered.

A more fundamental problem is how a free body in space can be stabilized. Since there are 12 degrees of freedom, 12 restraints are necessary logically. Fuller[5] shows that a bicycle wheel needs at least 12 spokes to stabilize its hub and proves that 12 restraints are necessary to fix a point in space (Fig. 3). Like a tent secured by its guy ropes, no additional tethers are necessary regardless of how the wind blows. Once rigidly fixed in space, external forces may change the magnitude but not the direction of the vectors.

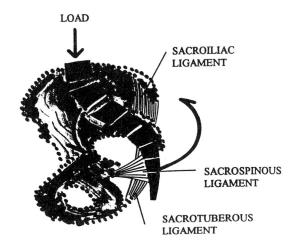

LOAD

SACROILIAC
LIGAMENT

SACROSPINOUS
LIGAMENT

SACROTUBEROUS
LIGAMENT

FIGURE 4. Tension forces balancing the pelvis.

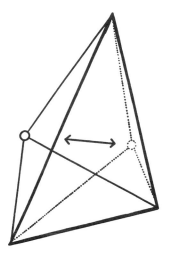

FIGURE 5. A body fixed in one plane by three tethers but still free to "piston" in the plane at right angles to the plane of the tethers. Twelve tethers oriented in the planes around the origin in a Cartesian coordinate system would keep the mass fixed at a point in space and not allow any translations or rotations.

What are the forces necessary to stabilize the sacrum? A sacrum has mass and, like a float in a parade, must be tethered to remain in place. The sacrum, tethered in three-dimensional space, can be rigidly restrained by 12 tension vectors. It would be suspended in the myofascial soft tissue network, like the hub of a wire bicycle wheel suspended by the spokes. Like the wire wheel, many additional "spokes" or tension elements can provide a fail-safe mechanism but confuse the picture a bit. Grant[6] and Kapandji[8] diagram the ligaments of the pelvis showing counterbalancing tension forces consistent with this concept (Fig. 4). The ligaments and myofascial components that attach to the pelvis must act as tension tethers, fixing the sacrum in its position in the body. Additional constraints, such as those discussed by Vleeming,[13] exist but may be species-specific and not a structural requirement. A wire wheel-modeled sacrum is omnidirectional and functions equally well when the load is applied from any direction. It depends on the intrinsic tension of the ligaments and muscles and not on gravity as a stabilizing force, in contrast to "keystone" and similar models. Since it does not depend on gravity to hold it in place, the sacrum functions equally well right side up, upside down, or sideways. A tension-fixed sacrum functions on land, in the air, at sea, or in a gravity free environment. It would work as the model for bipedal and quadrupedal stability and motion and, therefore, becomes the most widely adaptable of proposed models.

Like the hub of a wire wheel suspended by its spokes, the system must have a dynamic balance of the tension structures. A load on the wheel hub does not change the relative position of the hub within the rim. If the tension of the spokes remains constant, the hub does not move at all. Assuming a minimum of 12 properly vectored constraints, the hub is rigidly fixed. To move the hub, the opposing positive-negative spokes would need to be lengthened, shortened, or removed to allow the hub to move back and forth like a diaphragm (Fig. 5). To rotate the hub, the rim would need to be twisted; otherwise, twisting the hub will distort the rim (Fig. 6).

The rim must exert a counterforce equal and opposite to the tension forces pulling it to the hub. The subsystem of the wheel must integrate into the whole structure. The front wheel and rear wheel of a bicycle are linked together by a rigid frame that hangs from rims of the wheels like a swing suspended from its ropes. Because the link is rigid, twisting the front hub would create a twist on the rear hub.

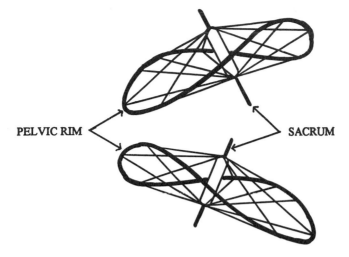

FIGURE 6.   Twisting the rim of a bicycle wheel forces the hub to tilt.

Therefore, the forces stabilizing the rear hub (the spokes) would stabilize the front hub also.

Ligaments of the body have high tensile strength[15] and would not distort much. The sacrum, as a hub, would move in harmony with the other bones of the pelvis, moving in and out like a diaphragm or rotating in a fixed relationship to the other bones. It is controlled by antagonistic muscles and by the tensile ligaments. For the most part, the ligaments have been ignored as prime movers in the body. Dorman[2] has proposed a clockwork mechanism in which the ligaments play a dynamic role in the walking cycle, with particular attention to the ligaments' role in pelvic mechanics. Stored energies in the ligaments are the torsion bars of the pelvis.

The double tie bar or four-bar hinge is the model for the dynamics of the cruciate ligament in the knee[3,11] (Fig. 7). The mechanism of a double tie bar hooked in series and the dynamic interaction of ligaments is apparent in a "Jacob's ladder," an ancient toy (Fig. 8). Flexing one rigid block creates a kinetic chain that sends all of the blocks in a controlled tumble, precisely organized by the controlling tension elements. These tension elements do not shorten or lengthen but, nevertheless, force the rigid blocks to move. If the end blocks are held so that tension is created through the system, the tumbling effect can move top to bottom, bottom to top, horizontally, or at any angle.

FIGURE 7.   Double tie bar knee. Positive rotation around the x axis of the femur ($+\theta$ x) creates an obligatory negative rotation around the x axis of the tibia ($-\theta$ x).

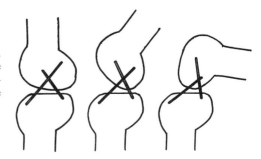

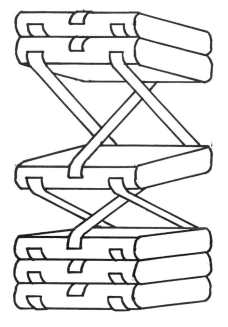

FIGURE 8.   Jacob's ladder. A crossed tie bar toy that demonstrates knee cruciate ligament action and serial interactions of a chain of tie bars.

In the spine, this type of movement has been described as coupled movement. Fryette[4] describes this movement in detail. However, the mechanical explanation for this movement pattern in the spine has been missing. If a double tie bar hinge exists in the spine, as it does in the knee, this coupling can be readily explained. The cruciate ligament arrangement is apparent in the microscopic and macroscopic organization of the annulus of the disk (Fig. 9). It is also seen in the three layers of transversospinales muscles and the costotransverse ligaments and the lumbar fascia. In this Jacob's ladder model of the spine, rotating the head or sacrum around the x, y

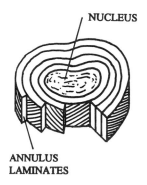

NUCLEUS

ANNULUS
LAMINATES

FIGURE 9.   Internal structure of a disk that demonstrates the crossed tie bar mechanism. (Adapted from White AA, Panjabi MM: Clinical Biomechanics of the Spine. Philadelphia, JB Lippincott, 1978.)

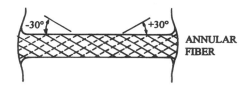

−30°   +30°

ANNULAR
FIBER

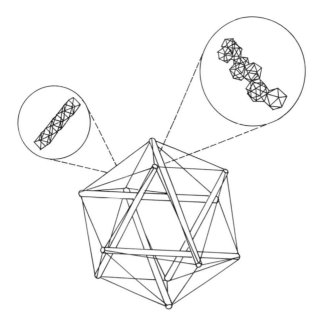

FIGURE 10.   Tension icosahedron. A hierarchical construct.

or z axis would create obligatory movements of the entire spine in a controlled pattern. The only actively contracting muscles (that could be seen by EMG studies) would be those needed to rotate the head or tail. The intrinsic tone of the ligaments and muscles of the disks and vertebrae controls the rest of the spine's movement.

When walking, the head tends to stay level and directed forward. It is the sacrum, wound by the counter-rotating ilia, that moves the spine. The vertical lift when walking imparts potential energy stored in the ligaments of the twisting ilia that then becomes the kinetic energy that powers the sacrum. As pointed out by Gracovetsky[7] and Dorman,[2] the limbs are propelled out from the central core like the arms of a vertical pendulum or a tetherball being unwound and rewound around its pole. Tension in the ligaments and muscles, preset like the spokes of a bicycle wheel, control both the stability and the movement pattern of the "spinal engine" described by Gracovetsky.[7]

Wire wheel-like structures have been termed "tensegrity" (for *tension integrity*) by Buckminster Fuller.[5] This is a class of constructs in which the compression elements, the rim and the hub (the wire wheel pelvis and the Jacob's ladder spine), are separated from are each other by tension elements and transmit the forces between them through these elements. According to Fuller,[5] the compressional "islands" are interpositioned in structural stability only by the tensional spokes. "Tension is primary and comprehensive, and compression is secondary and local." The tensegrity icosahedron is used by Wang et al.[14] as the model for cell structure (Fig. 10). Levin[9] proposes that the tension icosahedron is the primordial biomechanical structure. Tension elements coming from its 12 vertices would rigidly tether a central hub. The bones would be compression islands fixed in a tension network. A hierarchical system of tension icosahedrons is used by Levin[10] to model both the statics and dynamics of the body efficiently, with least energy costs.

Using this model, the sacrum is fixed in three-dimensional space because it is part of an integrated tensegrity structural system. Although the relationships between it and other bones remain fixed, it also moves. It may control the movement of the other bones in movement patterns such as walking, just as the front wheel of a bicycle affects the rear wheel. It may be the central force in these movements, the *Chi* in the ancient Chinese concept.

CONCLUSION

A new model for sacral mechanics is proposed that is consistent with mechanical laws and observed anatomic function and accounts for both the statics and dynamics of the sacrum in vertebrates. The sacrum is viewed as the hub of a tension network: the model provides for stability of the sacrum when it is loaded from any direction and can be used during bipedal or quadrupedal standing and walking or even standing on ones' head. Since the system requires low energy, it is favored by nature. This sacral model is consistent with a previously proposed integrated systems model of biomechanics.[9,10]

REFERENCES

1. Buczek FL, Kepple TM, Siegel KL, Stanhope SJ: Translational and rotational joint power terms in a six degree-of-freedom model of the normal ankle complex. J Biomech 27:1447–1457, 1994.
2. Dorman TA: Storage and release of elastic energy in the pelvis: Dysfunction, diagnoses and treatment. In Vleeming A, Mooney V, Snijders C, Dorman TA (eds): Low Back Pain and its Relation to the Sacroiliac Joint, Rotterdam, ECO, 1992, pp 586–600.
3. Dye SF: An evolutionary perspective of the knee. J Bone Joint Surg 69A:976–983, 1987.
4. Fryette HH: Principles of Osteopathic Technic. Colorado Springs, CO, American Acaedemy of Osteopathy, 1954.
5. Fuller RB: Synergetics. New York, Macmillian, 1975.
6. Grant JCB: A Method of Anatomy. Baltimore, Williams & Wilkins, 1952.
7. Gracovetsky S: The Spinal Engine. New York, Springer-Verlag, 1988.
8. Kapandji IA: The Physiology of Joints. New York, Churchill Livingstone, 1974.
9. Levin SM: The icosahedron as the three-dimensional finite element in biomechanical support. In Proceedings of the Society of General Systems Research Symposium on Mental Images, Values and Reality (Philadelphia,1986). St. Louis, Society of General Systems Research, 1986, pp G14–G26.
10. Levin SM: The primordial structure. In Banathy BH, Banathy BB (eds): Proceedings of the 34th annual meeting of the International Society for the Systems Sciences, Vol 2, Portland, OR, 1990, pp 716–720.
11. Muller W: The Knee. Form, Function and Ligament Reconstruction. New York, Springer, 1983.
12. Thompson D: On Growth and Form. London, Cambridge University Press, 1965.
13. Vleeming A, Volkers ACW, Snijders CJ, Stoeckart R: Relation between form and function in the sacroiliac joint: Part II: Biomechanical aspects. Spine 15:133–135, 1990.
14. Wang N, Butler JP, Ingber DE: Microtransduction across the cell surface and through the cytoskeleton. Science 260:1124–1127, 1993.
15. White AA, Panjabi MM: Clinical Biomechanics of the Spine. Philadelphia, JB Lippincott, 1978.
16. Woltring HJ: 3-D attitude representation of human joints: A standardization proposal. J Biomech 27:1399–1414, 1994.

HOWARD J. DANANBERG, DPM, FACFAOM

LOWER EXTREMITY MECHANICS AND THEIR EFFECT ON LUMBOSACRAL FUNCTION

From the Bedford Podiatry Group
The Walking Clinic
Bedford, New Hampshire

Reprint requests to:
Howard J. Dananberg, DPM,
  FACFAOM
Bedford Podiatry Group
The Walking Clinic
21 Eastman Avenue
Bedford, NH 03110-6701

Four-legged, apelike creatures evolved into the more upright, bipedal ancestors of humans millions of years ago. The trail left by their fossils demonstrates some of the subtle changes that took place. Simply standing erect was an option even for the earliest primates. Efficient forward movement during a period of single limb support, however, demanded significant changes within the structure and mechanics of the lower extremity, particularly the foot. A loosely aligned, gripping foot with long, plantarflexing digits evolved into a tightly compressed and therefore stable, yet pivotally oriented foot with shorter, dorsiflexing digits.[27] The ability to raise the center of the body over and beyond a single weightbearing limb provided an advantage that eventually permitted an increasingly stable upright posture.

Although the precise nature of the evolutionary course of humans is somewhat controversial, certain aspects are generally accepted. Approximately 3 million years ago, *Australopithecus afarensis*, or "Lucy," roamed Africa. Despite new features that permitted a more upright gait, Lucy retained many qualities that gave her a rather hunched, apelike appearance. Approximately 1.8 million years ago, two new predecessors evolved. *Panarthropus robustus*, although more upright, maintained an awkward, lumbering gait, whereas *Homo habilis* displayed a more advanced, erect style of walking. Both showed evidence of tool-making abilities and organized activities, yet *P. robustus* became extinct and *H. habilis* evolved into the human species. *H.*

SPINE: State of the Art Reviews—Vol. 9, No. 2, May 1995
Philadelphia, Hanley & Belfus, Inc.

389

habilis demonstrated a startling new property: the first metatarsal head had undergone a simple yet profound change in shape, structure, and function. It allowed dorsiflexion during loading and simultaneously created a closed-packed orientation (the stabilized position brought about by compression across the foot joints). In other words, *H. habilis* could step beyond the foot of the weightbearing limb and concurrently resist the applied forces in a mechanically efficient manner.

The ability to dorsiflex freely at the metatarsophalangeal joint during loading is a distinctly human trait. This motion is crucial to proper mechanics of the lower limbs and proper function of the erect lumbosacral structure.[9] The failure of this simple yet profound action has a pronounced effect on the low back. Understanding its pathomechanical influence, therefore, may alter clinical philosophy and improve results of treatment for chronic lower back pain. Dananberg, Lawton, et al.[13,22] reviewed a group of patients with chronic postural pain who had failed prior treatment and were considered at or near medical endpoint. After objective gait analysis and treatment with foot orthotics specifically designed to alter first metatarsophalangeal mechanics, 77% demonstrated 50–100% improvement over a 2-year period.

This chapter presents a new model for understanding the mechanics of human gait as well as the intricate interrelationships of the structures of the lower limbs. A description of functional hallux limitus—a common but locally asymptomatic primary pathomechanical process within the foot—forms the basis for understanding how gait mechanics cause stress to the lower back through repetitive motion injury. In addition, functional hallux limitus may be related directly to the high rate of repeat complaints in patients with lower back pain. Recognition that painful entities such as degenerative joint disease, disk herniation, and myogenic pain may result from a gait-related process of repetitive motion rather than primary, idiopathic disorders provides an improved model for evaluating patients. Also discussed are objective studies that support the beneficial effects of foot treatment on the more proximal joints and structures.

A NEW MODEL FOR LOWER LIMB FUNCTION DURING GAIT

In the classic view of human ambulation,[20] muscular action causes force moments across joints, which then create motion. However, careful examination of data related to phasic muscular contraction in the fully weightbearing lower limb fails to support this concept. Winter et al.[29] demonstrated that the majority of muscle contraction is of the eccentric type, which is 1.5–6 times stronger than concentric or shortening contraction.[1,3] Use of eccentric contraction is thus consistent with the concept that biologic action follows the most energy-conserving mode.

Yet the primary action of muscle during gait is to resist motion. How can the same muscle simultaneously resist and create motion? Obviously it cannot. Action of the weightbearing musculature, in coordination with the fascia and ligamentous structures within the lower limb, stabilizes joints at the foot, ankle, knee, and hip via the tensegrity model.[17,22] As the muscles resist lengthening, the increasing tension stabilizes the weightbearing limb to the physical forces applied during single limb support. The same muscular action, when relaxed, permits the stabilized joints to become flexible and thus enables their motion during swing phase. As the joints are stabilized, simultaneous loading provides elastic energy storage. Force is applied to the now resisting muscles, tendons, and ligaments and stored within them during heel strike to full-load phase, with simultaneous preparation for recoil during the second half of the step. In essence, gravity (through heel strike) provides the load that winds the spring. Recoil of this energy helps to move segments of the limb

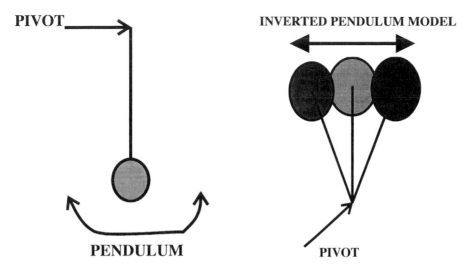

FIGURE 1.   *Left*, a pendulum suspended from a fixed, pivotal point swings back and forth under the influence of gravity. *Right*, an inverted pendulum model has been used to describe the relationship between the pelvis and lower extremity. The fixed pivotal point is located beneath the device that is in motion. As the spheres (representing the pelvis) advance from left to right, the relative position of the rod (representing the lower extremity and its connection at the hip) changes from flexed to extended position. This, in essence, is how the hip extends from under the torso during walking. It is the forward motion of the pelvis over the pivotal location provided by the foot.

during the power portion of the step.[2] This action is coordinated with additional input of energy, which is necessary to maintain consistent walking speed.[18]

When the ipsilateral limb is engaged in support, the contralateral limb performs the swing phase of motion. Instead of a simple catch-up action, the swing limb creates a centrifugal force that acts on the center of body mass. Thus swing phase has been viewed as pull phase.[7] Its action is sufficient to move the center of the body up and over the ipsilateral limb.[24] Once the center of body mass has advanced beyond the weightbearing limb, the effect of gravity continues to pull it toward the ground. Power from one side acts on the other, taking advantage of gravitational pull. The cycle is repeated from side to side[24] (Fig. 1).

Bipedal, erect gait requires that the torso, head, and neck must remain in a vertical position as the legs ambulate. In essence, the torso is pulled forward yet permitted to stay erect as the hip joint simultaneously rotates, allowing the supporting limb to move forward beneath it. Because the torso must move beyond the planted foot during single limb support, a comparable direction of rotation must be available at the point of foot-to-ground contact. This rotation is accomplished by action at three specific sites: (1) the round underside of the calcaneus; (2) the ankle joint, which can dorsiflex 10° beyond a right angle while loaded; and, most importantly, (3) the metatarsophalangeal joints, which also are capable of dorsiflexion during loading.[25] These pedal rotation sites are crucial to the efficient, functional coordination of the entire body. Without the ability to pivot the foot, extension at the hip joint during single limb support becomes impossible. When a person attempts to walk forward while wearing swimming fins, the awkward gait is related directly to the failure to pivot at the weightbearing foot (Figs. 2 and 3).

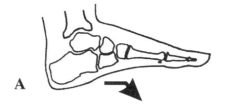

A

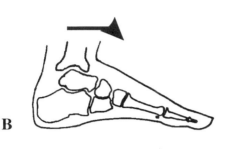

B

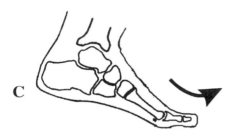

C

FIGURE 2. *A*, as the heel contacts the ground, the relatively round underside of the calcaneus permits forward rotation and the foot comes to full ground contact. *B*, once in full ground contact, the ankle joint dorsiflexes 10°, permitting the continued advancement of the body and simultaneously storing energy to create the next plantarflexion motion. *C*, the metatarsophalangeal joints provide the final pivotal site via dorsiflexion, permitting the heel to rise from the ground and advance over the fixed digits. These three sites form the pivotal motion of the foot necessary for forward ambulation.

The central feature of the various aspects of gait is their intercoordination. Each aspect depends on another to facilitate the process of walking. Central to this thesis is the factor that separated *P. robustus* from *H. habilis:* the closed packing stability related to the sagittal-plane pivot function of the foot. Although both had a hip joint capable of sagittal-plane motion, *P. robustus* lacked the concurrent ground pivot. Over the last 1.8 million years, evolutionary improvements in these interrelated motions led to the sophistication of human upright gait.

INTEGRATED FUNCTION OF THE LOWER LIMB, PELVIS, AND SPINE

Anatomic Review of the Foot

The human foot is a unique structure in the animal kingdom. It consists of 26 bones, each interdependent on the others for proper action. Its basic design has two functions: (1) to act initially as a loosely packed, adaptive structure capable of accumulating energy at heel strike and (2) to reverse this function with simultaneous compression, which grants stability. Both functions are necessary to permit forward motion. The foot and ankle may be divided into five separate components that function interdependently: (1) ankle joint (tibia-fibula-talor dome component), (2) subtalar joint, (3) midtarsal joints, (4) digits, and (5) metatarsophalangeal joints.

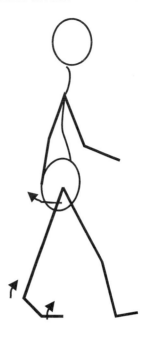

FIGURE 3.   Anatomic view of the hip joint extending from under the torso. The hip joint pivots through extension as the heel rises from the ground and pivots about the dorsiflexing metatarsophalangeal joints. Because gluteal action is shut off by midstance, the affect of the pull of the swing limb over the pivoting foot joints provides normal hip extension during walking.

TIBIA-FIBULA-TALAR DOME COMPONENT (ANKLE JOINT)

The distal tibia, distal fibula, and talar dome unite to form the ankle joint. Ligaments are present both medially and laterally as well as posteriorly. Forward stability of the talar dome depends on its articulation with the navicular bone, which possesses its own ligamentous structure.

The strong ligamentous structure between the tibia and fibula is known as the syndosmosis. Although the syndosmosis maintains taut structural integrity between the medial and lateral ankle structures, the ability of its fibers to reorient themselves allows some motion between the two bones.

The talar dome is covered with hyaline cartilage that permits smooth articulation with its concave counterpart on the distal tibia. The dome is shaped like a truncated pyramid, wider anteriorly than posteriorly. Therefore, as the ankle joint dorsiflexes, the wider portion of the dome must fit between the tibial and fibular components of the proximal aspect of the ankle. To facilitate this motion, the fibular component is capable of a lateral-upward translation. The orientation of the syndosmotic fibers is initially oblique, but they move to a tighter, horizontal position as the fibula translates with ankle dorsiflexion. These motions also serve to move toward closed-packed foot alignment, which becomes necessary as the body rapidly advances up and over the foot, and to store energy that assists in the ensuing plantarflexion of the ankle.

SUBTALAR JOINT

The plantar surface of the talus contains three joint surfaces that correspond to the dorsal surface of the calcaneus: the anterior, middle, and posterior facets of the subtalar joint. The motion within this series of joints occurs in unison and has been described as screwlike because it is multidirectional in specific combinations. (A screw moves downward while turning clockwise and upward while turning counterclockwise.) This screwlike quality permits two directionally predetermined, triplanar forms of motion: supination and pronation. The supinatory motion includes inversion, plantarflexion, and adduction, whereas the pronatory motion includes eversion, dorsiflexion, and abduction. Both the medial and lateral aspects of the joints are stabilized by strong external ligaments as well as by an array of internal ligaments that line the canal (sinus tarsi) between the talus and calcaneus. This canal lies along the axis of motion of the subtalar joint and is rich in mechanoreceptors.

In some ways, the subtalar joint may be viewed as a differential gear. It is capable of converting the internal and external limb rotations to pronation and supination of the foot. When forced into load during heel strike, the subtalar joint pronates. The talus migrates medially as the calcaneus counterrotates beneath it. This pattern of motion coordinates with the internal rotation of the tibia, femur, and pelvis directly above. As the initial impact approaches its peak load, the center of body mass is pulled forward by the initiating swing phase of the opposite limb. The foot of the weightbearing limb must manage increasing loads as the center of the body advances over it. The enabling mechanism is a reversal of action: the limb that rotated internally at impact now rotates externally as the opposite limb pulls forward and rotates the pelvis through the transverse plane. Simultaneously the subtalar joint moves from pronation to supination, which coordinates with external rotation from above. This sequence is facilitated by ligamentous storage of energy at heel strike as well as other actions described below.

MIDTARSAL JOINTS

The midtarsal joints consist of a series of bones (navicular, cuboid, and three cuneiforms) that function as a junction between the ankle/subtalar complex and the sagittal plane motion of the metatarsophalangeal joints. They also serve as attachments to all or part of the posterior tibial, anterior tibial, or peroneus longus muscles. Strong ligamentous connections permit limited but necessary motions among the midtarsal joints as well as closed-packed alignment when increasing loads are applied.

DIGITS

Each foot has five digits. The great toe has a single interphalangeal joint, whereas the four lesser toes have two. The increased size and unique anatomy of the great toe relate to specific functional requirements (discussed below) during gait. The toes are the only structures specifically designed to be stationary during the single support phase. The toenails, which cover the distal dorsal portions, are quite strong and do not deform significantly during loading. At their origin on the dorsum of the distal phalanx, the flexor tendons, which normally are plantar oriented, send slips that attach directly into the dorsal nail roots or matrix and act as a bridle, stabilizing the digits from above and maintaining their role as anchors.

METATARSOPHALANGEAL JOINTS

The metatarsophalangeal joints are highly specialized to permit bipedal ambulation in the erect human. While loaded, they allow the full-range dorsiflexion necessary for forward movement. In addition, their integrated design with the fascia maintains the closed-packed orientation of the more proximal aspects of the foot and limb. Because of its significance in normal function, the great toe is described in detail.

The great toe joint (the first metatarsophalangeal joint) consists of the head of the first metatarsal, tibial, and fibular sesamoids and the base of the proximal phalanx. The first metatarsal head is situated, like a body lying in a hammock, within the thick capsular wall formed on the medial, lateral, and inferior surfaces. It is stable when located in the center, because the capsular wall maintains its position. When it moves or rotates too far medially, it loses the stability of the capsular wall and dislocation results (hallux valgus). The first metatarsal joint has no tendinous attachments at its distal end. At its proximal end, the peroneus longus attaches to the medial cuneiform. The base of the proximal phalanx, however, has tendinous attachments on four sides: the abductor hallucis (medially), both heads of the adductor hallucis (laterally), the extensor hallucis longus (dorsally via the hood apparatus), and the tendons of the flexor hallucis brevis (plantarly). In addition, 50% of the entire thickness of the plantar aponeurosis is attached to the plantar base of the proximal phalanx of the great toe. The plantar aponeurosis also sends attachments to the plantar fat pad directly under the metatarsal heads. The remaining half of the plantar aponeurosis attaches into the base of each of the lesser digits, with a progressively decreasing thickness laterally. This arrangement provides a fixed platform and allows the toes and fat pad to serve as a buttress against the mobile metatarsal heads.[4]

The freely mobile metatarsal heads provide a pivotal foundation about which the advancing body can move. The base of each metatarsal travels up and over the weightbearing heads. The fat pad, located directly under each metatarsal head, provides a relatively friction-free surface because of its oily consistency. The digits serve as a buttress, preventing the metatarsals from sliding forward and encouraging proper rotation when the heel elevates as the body advances.

The motion of the first metatarsophalangeal, which is a ginglymoarthrodial joint, is unique; it uses both hinge and gliding action to achieve its full range. At heel lift direct hinge action between the proximal phalanx and the first metatarsal accounts for approximately 20°. The first metatarsal accounts for about 45° as it glides in a plantarflexion-eversion direction over the sesamoid apparatus for the remainder of the step. Thus the total available range of motion is about 65°, which is required for normal movement of the torso and leg. During single support phase, the hip joint extends on the torso for a maximum of 20°; a comparable site must be available at the foot-to-ground contact. Once contralateral heel strike occurs, the ipsilateral leg changes its direction of motion; it begins to flex at both the knee and hip and to plantarflex at the ankle. Because 20° of ankle plantarflexion and 45° of knee flexion are necessary to achieve the correct position at toe-off, a comparable amount of dorsiflexion must be achieved at the metatarsophalangeal joint. Hence the total available range of motion is 65°.[26]

Integrated Foot and Limb Function

Motion of the lower extremity joints during the gait cycle is summarized in Table 1. Hicks described the foot as a structure in which each bone is capable of rotating in a direction opposite to adjacent bones.[19] Thus a series of articulations reverses the motion of the bones as they are loaded and unloaded. This property of "left- and right-handedness" has a distinct advantage, as exemplified in the reverse actions of the ankle and metatarsophalangeal joints. As one moves in a particular direction, the other moves in the opposite direction. Such actions are necessary because of the opposing structural alignment between the upright limb and horizontal foot. The knee and hip also fit within the reverse paradigm: when one is extended, the other is flexed. As the knee extends, its posterior aspect widens. In the hip, however, extension widens the anterior surface but narrows the posterior aspect. Reverse

TABLE 1.   Motion of the Lower Extremity Joints

Joint	Initial Double Support	Initial Single Support	Terminal Single Support	Terminal Double Support
Hip joint	Initial flexion, then extension	Extension	Fully extended	Rapid flexion
Knee joint	Flexion, then extension	Extension	Fully extended	Rapid flexion
Ankle joint	Initial plantar-flexion, then dorsiflexion	Dorsiflexion	Plantarflexion	Rapid plantarflexion
Metatarso-phalangeal joints	Initial dorsiflexion, then neutral	Neutral	Dorsiflexion	Rapid dorsiflexion

actions create stability, store energy, and simultaneously allow one limb to use the pull force of the contralateral limb for forward motion.

The concept of closed packing was described by Bosjen-Möller in 1979.[5] The ability to compress the calcaneal-cuboid joint at a specific point in the step completely stabilizes the foot via a weight shift across the lateral to medial forefoot. This shift rapidly increases tension within the plantar aponeurosis. The stable foot can be lifted from the heel, rotating forward about the metatarsal heads as the metatarsophalangeal joints dorsiflex. The attachment of the aponeurosis to the base of the proximal phalanx progressively tightens, pulling the calcaneus (the origin of the aponeurosis) toward the metatarsal heads. The increasing tension, explained by the tensegrity model, enhances stability as the advancing body causes exponential increases in the loading of the foot. This tightening of the aponeurosis also causes the subtalar to supinate via the windlass mechanism and therefore to accommodate the external rotation within the weightbearing femur and tibia.

The progressive tightening within the aponeurosis across the plantar surface of the foot can be likened to loading a sling shot. The sesamoid apparatus, like the projectile loaded in the sling, releases and projects the foot forward as it enters the final stages of the toe-off phase.[14] Although this action cannot directly move the entire body forward, it adds impetus to the initiation of swing phase, which in turn provides its own pulling force.

Developing Swing-Phase Motion

As the contralateral swing limb develops a pulling force, rotations of the ipsilateral hip (extension) and foot (dorsiflexion of the metatarsophalangeal joints) permit the weightbearing femur to extend from under the torso during single support. This action can be viewed as a "preload" to the next swing phase. Like a cocked gun, it is ready to be released in coordination with the elastic return concurrently created with the pelvis.

As energy is released from the spine (see chapter 6), the pelvis begins a forward rotation about the ipsilateral hip. This action coordinates with contralateral heel strike. The trailing ipsilateral leg has just reached full extension at the hip and knee joints. At this moment, the support musculature of the trailing limb is turned off, "collapsing" the limb. The hip and knee immediately reverse into rapid flexion, accompanied by plantarflexion of the ankle and dorsiflexion of the metatarsophalangeal joints. This quick reversal creates a rapid, forward acceleration of the femur, which is the initial action of swing-phase motion. Once it has accelerated to a point

THE EFFECT OF FUNCTIONAL HALLUX LIMITUS

FIGURE 4. *A*, as the body advances, it attempts to lift the heel from the ground by pivoting about the metatarsophalangeal joints. *B*, the sagittal blockade of functional hallux limitus causes the midtarsal joint to provide some of the lost sagittal plane motion. This is visible as late midstance pronation with marked lowering of the medial longitudinal arch. Other manners of compensation exist throughout the more proximal joint (see Figs. 6 and 7).

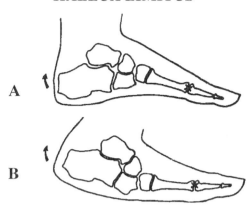

directly beneath the torso, an energy-returning toe-off occurs, accompanied by a burst of the iliopsoas musculature (primary hip flexors) designed to perpetuate (rather than simply generate) the swing-phase motion. The limb kicks outward and pulls on the center of the body. Each step repeats this cycle.[12]

UNDERSTANDING THE ABNORMAL GAIT PROCESS

Functional Hallux Limitus

Functional hallux limitus represents a contradiction between findings during clinical examination and findings during gait. In a classic, non-weightbearing examination of the foot, the first metatarsophalangeal joint may demonstrate full, non-painful range of motion. During the single support, full weightbearing portion of gait, however, no range of motion is found. This paradox defines functional hallux limitus. The first metatarsophalangeal joint fails both to provide the pivotal site required for forward motion and to create the closed-packed alignment necessary for stabilization as progressive loads are applied during gait. The patient rarely exhibits symptoms of pain or swelling in the first metatarsophalangeal joint and is unaware of any other problem that may reflect its involvement in abnormal gait[9,11,28] (Fig. 4).

Normally, the pull exerted on the center of body mass creates motion over the supporting foot as the weightbearing limb extends from under the torso. Because this process requires the foot to provide a sagitally oriented pivotal site, failure to develop this pivot is visible at the various sites at which the force must be dissipated. Because the total power input for any step (pull, momentum, gravity, elastic energy return) must be equivalent to the total body weight to maintain speed of gait, the aggregate amount of energy to be dissipated is quite significant. When compensatory motions occur over time (40–70 million times/decade), they have a substantial effect on postural integrity, as the axiom "form follows function" dictates (Figs. 5, 6, and 7).

Many forms of gait are common, including abducted or "duck-foot" vs. adducted or "pigeon-toe" positions, straight vs. flexed knee, normal lordosis vs. straight back, and erect vs. hunched posture. Common belief relates these "forms" to individual anatomic variation or to a painful process such as limping secondary to

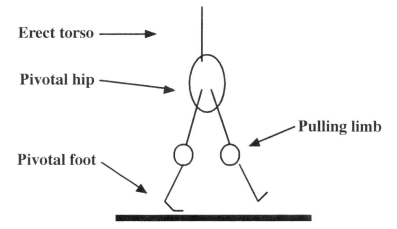

FIGURE 5.   The pull limb causes the trailing limb to extend at the hip joint provided the foot provides a pivotal site about which the body can advance.

injury. In fact, however, such forms often progress over a lifetime and precede the painful process. For instance, the hunched appearance of an 80-year-old patient is neither spontaneous nor congenital. It is a slow process that takes place over a long period. A careful evaluation of the patient's gait (long before the final form develops) may provide subtle clues to the motions (functions) that eventually result in postural deterioration (form).

Wolfe's law, proposed in the late nineteenth century, clearly describes this phenomenon, which is disguised by its slow rate of development and subtle nature. Although specific congenital or acute trauma-induced changes may cause some of the classic postures of patients with chronic low back pain, loss of motion in the first metatarsophalangeal joint may be partially or totally responsible and/or act as a per-

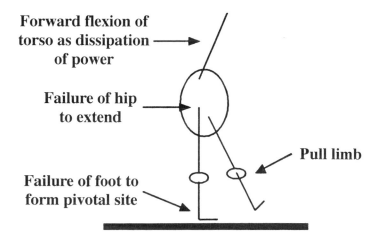

FIGURE 6.   The limb fails to achieve full extension secondary to the loss of pivot of the foot. Power dissipation causes the torso to flex forward as it continues to be pulled forward by the swinging limb.

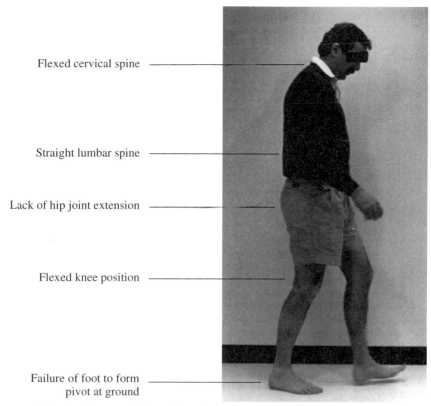

Flexed cervical spine

Straight lumbar spine

Lack of hip joint extension

Flexed knee position

Failure of foot to form
pivot at ground

The classic postural form of a patient with functional hallux limitus

FIGURE 7. "Form follows function" is an axiom described by Julius Wolfe at the end of the nineteenth century. Although well understood in some contexts, the poor posture of a middle-aged adult is not viewed according to this axiom. Once the effect of sagittal plane blockade at the foot level is understood, this structural alignment can be seen as a postural change (form) related to style of gait (function).

petuating factor. Because motion at the first metatarsophalangeal joint is visible only when the heel is lifted and pivoted over the joint, any block of joint motion that prevents heel lift hides the etiologic nature of functional hallux limitus. Other postural accommodations (Tables 2 and 3) have been assumed to be primary responses. Only in the context of functional hallux limitus is the secondary nature of their pathomechanics understood. Failure to identify functional hallux limitus leads to the perpetuation of improper motions and their associated complaints.

Lumbosacral Stress Associated with Functional Hallux Limitus

The tensegrity model describes support of the lumbosacral region through coordination of compression in osseous structures and tension in soft tissues.[23] These support also depends on the position of the various structures at specific times of load application. Failure of osseous and soft-tissue structures to achieve their appropriate position may be related directly to the presence of functional hallux limitus

TABLE 2. Direct Sagittal Plane Compensation for Functional Hallux Limitus

Specific Joint	Segment of Stance Phase	Normal Motion	Compensatory Motion
Midtarsal joint	Midstance	Supination (arch raising)	Pronation (arch lowering)
Ankle joint	Midstance through toe-off	Plantarflexion	Dorsiflexion
Knee joint	Midstance through opposite limb contact	Motion to complete extension	Failure to fully extend (knee remains flexed)
Hip joint	Single limb support	Full-range extension to 15–20°	Limited extension with failure to achieve 15–20°
Lumbar spine	Single limb support	Increasing lordosis (extension)	Forward flexion (straight back)
Cervical spine	Single limb support	Increasing lordosis (head erect)	Forward flexion (head down and forward)

and often leads to two specific pain patterns caused by diskogenic lumbar disorders and myogenic overuse. Myogenic overuse involves the iliopsoas, quadratus lumborum, and gluteus maximus-iliotibial band complex. Although described separately in this chapter, the two processes are connected closely and should not be viewed as completely separate events.

STRESS TO THE LUMBAR DISKS

Cumulative stress, even at relatively low levels, may weaken the structure of intervertebral disks over time.[15] At lower levels, the forces necessary to cause injury must include lateral bending and rotation as well as compressive loads. Magnetic resonance imaging often demonstrates marked desiccation of intervertebral disks as a sign of long-term stresses. The primary effect (95–97% of cases) is evident at the L4–L5 and L5–S1 intervertebral spaces.[16] The single event (e.g., bending, lifting-twisting) that results in frank disk prolapse and disability may be only the final incident in a longer series of microtraumatic events. Even when a herniated disk is detected and surgically removed, statistics show a high rate of recurrence within 4 years after treatment. This section demonstrates how subtle gait malfunction may be the hidden stressfull event that results in disk weakening. The events of a single step (lateral bending, rotation, and compression) may be repeated in excess of 2500 times/side/day.

The events that cause stress occur during two separate stages of the gait cycle. The initial compression load to the disk begins in the second half of the single support phase and concludes with the contralateral heel strike. Once the disk is placed under compression load, a lateral-bend, rotational force is applied as the ipsilateral limb moves from weightbearing to swing-phase motion. Lifting the limb into swing phase is equivalent to lifting approximately 15% of body weight. Failure to lift correctly applies bending/rotational stress directly to the L4–L5 and L5–S1 disks.[11]

TABLE 3. Avoidance Maneuvers for Functional Hallux Limitus

Normal Motion during Single Limb Support	Avoidance Motion during Single Limb Support
Rectus foot position	Abducted foot position
Rectus foot position	Adducted foot position
Heel off by 60% of stance phase	Heel off after 60% of stance phase (delayed heel off)
Propulsive toe-off	Vertical lift-off (thus avoiding full dorsiflexion of metatarsophalangeal joints)

Pathomechanical Events in the Gait Cycle as Related to Functional Hallux Limitus

ILIOPSOAS AND L4–L5, L5–S1 DISK STRESS

As the contralateral swing phase begins, the center of the body is pulled forward to a point directly above the ipsilateral weightbearing limb. At this point, the torso is erect, the hip joint is neutral, and the femur and tibia/fibula are aligned vertically. As the center of the body advances beyond this point, the heel is raised from the ground and the hip and metatarsophalangeal joints rotate clockwise, maintaining the torso in the erect position. The hip joint is visibly extended, and the thigh extends outward under the torso. Functional hallux limitus alters the results of energy input. Because functional hallux limitus blocks pivotal heel lift, the center of the body responds with the flexion compensation described in Table 2. This response creates a loss of lumbar lordosis by replacing extension with flexion. Lumbar flexion creates a posterior-directed compression on the disk, causing it to protrude against the nerve roots in the posterior aspect of the spine. By reducing the lordotic curve, flexion also spreads the lumbar facets. When aligned lordotically, the facets prevent side-bending and rotation of the lumbar spine.[21] When the facets are spread, however, osseous restriction of motion is lost. This loss becomes extremely important in the second phase of the process.[11]

Approximately 200 ms after the lumbar disks are stressed by flexion accommodation, contralateral heel strike occurs. The force of heel strike prepares the already compressed disk to be torqued when ipsilateral swing is initiated. As described above, swing phase may be initiated by the mechanism of extension preload. Functional hallux limitus adversely affects the ability to achieve full extension; instead, the limb fails to move from under the torso. As the limb is released to initiate swing phase, the femur drops down instead of accelerating forward. Therefore, the iliopsoas muscle (Fig. 8), which is designed to perpetuate the forward swinging of the limb, must stop its downward fall and initiate swing motion. This action eventually leads to localized tissue injury, because it is repeated thousands of times per day during normal ambulation. Symptoms of iliopsoas overuse include pain along the iliac crest, low spine, and, in later stages, groin; difficulty with flexing the hip is evident.[6]

The iliopsoas originates directly from the disks and intervertebral septa of Ll through L4. When the weight of the lower limb becomes sufficiently burdensome, the action of the iliopsoas affects its origin as much as its insertion. When the femur is fixed and the iliopsoas fires, the results are lateral flexion ipsilaterally and rotation contralaterally.[20] Because these actions are brought about via the insertion of Ll–L4, they function as a piston directly over the L5–Sl vertebra and are consistent with the high levels of microtraumatic events necessary for chronic degeneration. Symptoms from such stress may include classic radicular complaints, such as sciatic radiational pain or other symptoms related to nerve root compression.

ADDITIONAL MYOGENIC BACK PAIN AND LATERAL HIP PAIN

Analysis of the swing phase of motion has been shown to be one of the few constants in the evaluation of the gait of a neurologically normal subject.[8] The angular displacements and muscle firing sequences for the hip, knee, and ankle are strikingly similar throughout the population. Even newborn infants, when held erect by their arms, exhibit the swing-phase reflex, which appears to have input from the nervous system regardless of the position from which it originates. Since the time at

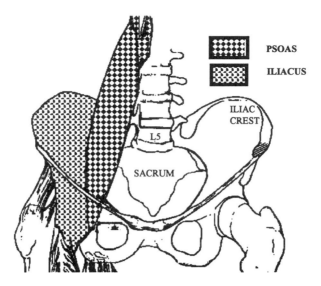

FIGURE 8. The psoas muscle originates from L1–L4, the intervertebral septa, and disks. The iliacus originates from the iliac crest. They insert into the lessor trochanter of the medial femur and fire at toe-off to flex the thigh on the pelvis. Strain during limb lift eventually produces overuse symptoms of these muscles as well as pain at their site of origin.

which swing phase initiates appears relatively fixed as related to gait speed, the position from which this motion will begin becomes critically important. Failure to achieve appropriate extension at the hip joint prior to swing initiation creates a functionally deficient and therefore stressful anatomic alignment from which to begin this activity. The repetitive nature of this action becomes the pathogenesis for lumbar distress.

Lateral trunk bending appears to be universally effective at initiating swing phase when the trailing limb is poorly positioned. This mechanism uses the torso to drag the trailing limb into motion. Once this action begins, hip flexion and knee extension occur on their own. When repeated as a gait habit thousands of times per day, however, the lateral trunk bend eventually leads to an additional series of complaints in patients with chronic lower back pain.[12]

The timing of the trunk bend correlates with the onset of contralateral heel strike. Because of limited hip extension, the ipsilateral limb is poorly positioned to initiate the next swing phase; thus the trunk begins an ipsilateral-to-contralateral motion to achieve maximal bend at the moment of toe-off. The structures that appear to be directly related to this action are the contralateral gluteus maximus/iliotibial band complex and the contralateral quadratus lumborum. Once ipsilateral toe-off occurs, the trunk immediately returns to a rectus position. Symptoms include back pain between the twelfth rib and iliac crest as well as acute tenderness over the length of the iliotibial band. Often complaints related to the iliotibial band are described by the patient as radiational and may be confused with radicular (sciatic) nerve radiation when in fact they are fascial in origin. Palpation of pain along the iliotibial band, even at its most distal aspect, helps to determine the nature of the complaint. Bursitis of the greater trochanteric joint also may be a symptom of this process. Symptoms are usually unilateral, but if both the ipsilateral and contralateral

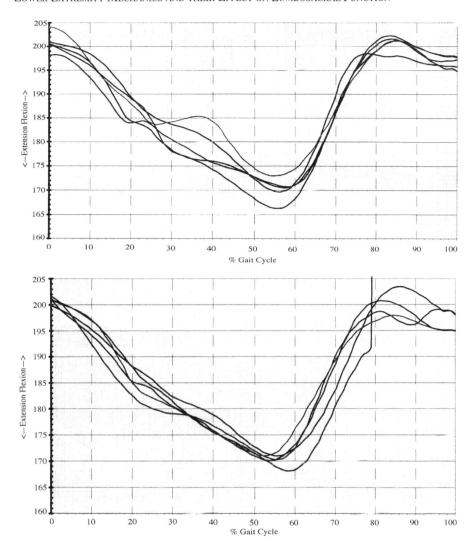

FIGURE 9. *A*, hip joint range of motion in a patient with low back pain without corrective orthotic devices. The vertical axis reflects flexion (increasing slope) and extension (downward slope), and the horizontal axis represents percentage of gait cycle. Each line demonstrates a single trial from a series of 30 trials. Note the variability between each of the lines. In two, a reversal of extension during single support phase is visible as the lines stop descending and flatten abruptly. *B*, hip joint range of motion in the same patient but with corrective orthotic devices. Note the symmetry among the five trials. The previous restriction to hip extension has been replaced with progressive motion in the correct direction. Symptoms completely resolved.

limbs exhibit poor hip extension mechanics and trunk bending is necessitated in both directions, they certainly may be bilateral. Radicular complaints also may be associated with trunk bending. Because the quadratus lumborum inserts not only into the iliac crest but also into the inferior iliolumbar ligament, repeated lateral

se rotational moment on the fifth lumbar vertebra. In patients with
\sition during midstance, the spread of the posterior vertebral facets
osseous stability against excessive rotation, and nerve root stress

FOOT ORTHOTICS AND POSTURAL MOTION

Discussion of examination for and fabrication of foot orthotics is beyond the scope of this chapter. The crucial point is the beneficial effect of properly fitted orthotics on postural pain, as evidenced by studies of how they alter total extension of the hip. Figure 9 depicts before-and-after series of hip joint extension in one patient. Subjects walked across a 30' x 6' gait platform for 30 passes, wearing only shoes, and were filmed with reflective markers on the hips, knees, and ankles. After completion of the first trial, they placed in their shoes custom foot orthotics designed specifically to treat functional hallux limitus (Kinetic Wedge Orthotic, Langer Biomechanics Group, Deer Park, N.Y.) and walked for 30 additional passes. Trials were repeated without and then with orthotics. The two figures show the 5th, 10th, 15th, 20th, and 25th pass both with and without orthotics. The consistency of hip extension with orthotics is clearly demonstrated. When the hip is permitted to extend adequately from under the torso, swing-phase motion is efficient. Stress to the lumbar spine is reduced, as is the need for lateral trunk bending.

CONCLUSION

In chronic low back pain, patients do not limp because they hurt,
but rather hurt because they limp.

Human evolution appears to be significantly related to development of erect, two-legged ambulation. Major changes within the lower extremity permitted this advancement. Of all adaptations, the ability of the foot to serve as a pivotal point about which the entire body can advance is of primary importance. The motions of the lumbosacral spine during normal walking depend on this function. With failure of sagittal plane mechanics within the foot, direct compensation and/or indirect stress must be applied to the lower back thousands of times per day. Tens of millions of destructive cycles over the years result in secondary degenerative changes. Recognizing the primary effect of abnormal gait on erect posture is essential in providing an effective treatment protocol. In a retrospective study, 77% of patients who had postural pain without foot symptoms and were considered at or near medical endpoint exhibited 50–100% improvement when functional hallux limitus was corrected with the appropriate foot orthotic.

REFERENCES

1. Abbott BD, Bigland B, Ritchie JM: The physiological cost of negative work. J Physiol (Lond) 117:380, 1952.
2. Alexander RM: The spring in your step. New Scientist April 30:42, 1987.
3. Banister EW, Brown SR: Relative energy requirements of physical activity. In Falls HB (ed): Exercise Physiology. New York, Academic Press, 1968.
4. Bosjen-Moller F: Calcaneocuboid joint and stability of the longitudinal arch of the foot at high and low gear push off. J Anat (Lond) 129:165–176, 1979.
5. Bosjen-Moller F, Lamoreux L: Significance of free dorsiflexion of the toes in walking. Acta Orthop Scand 50:471–479, 1979.
6. Cailliet R: Lower Back Pain Syndrome. 3rd ed. Philadelphia, FA Davis, 1974.
7. Claeys R: The analysis of ground reaction forces in pathologic gait. Int Orthop 113–119, 1993.
8. Cook T, Cozzens B: Human solutions for locomotion: The initiation of gait. In Herman R, et al (eds): Neural Control of Locomotion. New York, Plenum Press, 1976.

9. Dananberg HJ: Functional hallux limitus and its effect on normal ambulation. J Curr Podiatr Med 1985.
10. Dananberg HJ: Subtle gait malfunction and its effect on chronic musculoskeletal pain. J Orthop Med 1992.
11. Dananberg HJ: Gait style as an etiology to chronic postural pain. Part I: Functional hallux limitus. J Am Podiatr Med Assoc 83:433–441, 1993.
12. Dananberg HJ: Gait style as an etiology to chronic postural pain. Part II: The postural compensatory process. J Am Podiatr Med Assoc 83:615–624, 1993.
13. Dananberg HJ, DiNapoli DR, Lawton M: Hallux limitus and non-specific bodily trauma. In DiNapoli DR (ed): Reconstructive Surgery of the Foot. Tucker, GA, Podiatry Institute, 1990.
14. David R, Delagouttcc JP, Rinard M. Anatomical study of the sesamoid bones of the 1st metatarsal. J Am Podiatr Med Assoc 79:536–544, 1989.
15. Farfan HF, Cossette JW, Robertson GH, et al: The effects of torsion on the lumbar intervertebral joints: The role of torsion in the production of disc degeneration. J Bone Joint Surg 52A:468–497.
16. Farfan H, Kirkaldy-Willis WH: The present status of spinal fusion in the treatment of lumbar intervertebral joint disorders. Clin Orthop 158:98–124.
17. Fuller B: Synergetics. New York, Macmillan, 1975.
18. Gracovetsky S: The Spinal Engine. New York, Springer-Verlag, 1987.
19. Hicks JH: The mechanics of the foot. Part II: The plantar aponeurosis and the arch. J Anat (Lond) 25–30, 1954.
20. Inman et al: Human Walking. Baltimore, Williams & Wilkins, 1981.
21. Kapanji IA: The Physiology of the Joints, vol. 3, 2nd ed. Edinburgh, Churchill Livingstone, 1974.
22. Lawton M, Dananberg HJ: Functional hallux limitus and chronic musculoskeletal pain [abstract]. J Phys Med Rehabil 1991.
23. Levin S: The space truss as a model for cervical spine mechanics—a systems science concept. In Peterson J, Burn L (eds): Back Pain: An International Review. Boston, Kluwer, pp 231–238.
24. Mann RA, Moran GT, Dougherty SE: Muscle activity in running, jogging and sprinting. Am J Sport Med 14, 1968.
25. Perry J: Gait Analysis: Normal and Pathologic Function. Thorofare, NJ, Slack, 1992.
26. Root M, Weed J, Orien W, et al: Abnormal and Normal Function of the Foot. Los Angeles, Clinical Biomechanics Corp., 1977.
27. Susman R: Evolution of the human foot: Evidence from plio-pleistocene hominids. Foot Ankle 3:365–376, 1983.
28. Wernick J, Dananberg HJ: Secondary active retrograde pronation and the ideology to overuse injuries. Podiatry Tracts, 1988.
29. Winter DA, Scott S: Techniques for interpretation of electromyography for concentric and eccentric contractions in gait. J Electromyogr Kinesiol 1:263, 1991.

THOMAS A. DORMAN, MD
ANDRY VLEEMING, PhD

SELF-LOCKING OF THE SACROILIAC ARTICULATION

Private Practice
San Luis Obispo, California (TAD)
        and
Department of Anatomy
Erasmus University
Rotterdam
The Netherlands (AV)

This is an age of confidence in science. We suppose that the basics have been worked out. Since Isaac Newton defined the three laws of mechanics with *principia* more than 300 years ago, it is assumed that there is room only for refinements. Only a few variations and details of anatomy have been defined this century. It is therefore a shock to the comfort zone when contemporary researchers raise questions on form and function. Physicians and biologists should take note of physical scientists. Three centuries after Newton and almost a century after Einstein, questions are being raised about forces, about the time/space continuum, and about force-fields. Fundamental questions regarding form and function in biologic structures have been raised in sotto voce only now and again by Russell[19] and more poignantly by Thompson[26] earlier this century. This volume challenges some basic concepts about the transfer of forces within living organisms.[24] The paradox that hyaline cartilage is soft but able to withstand the seeming direct transfer of great loads in the living state is at the nub of the dilemma. This chapter will review recent research and present a new understanding of the function of the human sacroiliac joint from a reductionist point of view.

Active movement is a characteristic of the animal kingdom. In multicellular organisms it is accompanied by the "problem" of stability versus mobility. In the case of flagellae feathers and scales, elasticity with a cyclic wave form is known to occur. Vertebrates have solved the problem of mobility versus stability with the in-

SPINE: State of the Art Reviews—Vol. 9, No. 2, May 1995
Philadelphia, Hanley & Belfus, Inc.

407

vention of the joint; therefore, the study of *arthrology* is protean to the unique characteristic of all the genera concerned. A fundamental look at the transfer of forces in static structures will serve well as a prelude to an analysis of the interaction of tension members (ligaments and fascia) with compression members (bones and joints) in living organisms.

Prestressed reinforced concrete bears weight vertically in pillars and in cantilevered beams better than native amorphous concrete. When required to define the locus of the forces, structural engineers respond that the structures function as a whole. The simplistic analysis of seeing vertical supports intuitively as a pile of bricks, therefore, missed at least some of the point of how more weight is borne with less.

Living limbs do more than bear weight. Angulation and torsion forces are transferred through them as well as traction, torque integrated with other parts of the body. Therefore, the function of limbs is more complex than merely that of weight-bearing. It is not surprising, therefore, that lines of force, trabeculae, have been identified in bones, and it is since the research of Julius Wolff[37] that we have recognized the extraordinary property of living connective tissue to align itself appropriately for stress, the alignment of bony trabeculae in the human femur being the most familiar example. In modern times the alignment of fibroblasts in tissue culture has been observed[15] and is seemingly a cellular counterpart of what is now called Wolff's Law. Laws are merely groupings of observed phenomena in patterns; they are open to skepticism. Good science leads not only to more answers but also to better questions.

The importance of friction in the function of the sacroiliac joints has been conveyed through the introduction of the contrasting concepts of *form closure* and *force closure*.[27] Form closure refers to a stable situation with closely fitting joint surfaces. In an idealized model of form closure, weightbearing and the transfer of other forces would be achieved through snugly fitting geometrical forms alone. Functional analysis of living joints shows that various mechanical refinements are usually present in each. In the case of the sacroiliac joints, the additional factors are distinct. On first inspection the sacrum appears to be wedged between the ilia. However, on standing, the closed kinematic chain is predicated on lateral pressures through the rough surfaces of these joints. The term *force closure* applies here. In the sacroiliac joints both a compressive lateral force and friction are needed to withstand vertical loads. Shear at the sacroiliac joints is prevented by a combination of the specific anatomic features (form closure) and the compression generated by ligaments and muscles acting across the high friction surfaces (force closure). These concepts are represented in Figures 1 and 2.

THE SACROILIAC JOINTS

Anatomy

Two different aspects of roughening of the auricular surfaces of the sacroiliac joints were seen in a gross anatomic study of 47 specimens derived from the dissection room of Erasmus University in Rotterdam.[31] There was roughening in texture; ridges and depressions were observed. A classification of the degree of roughness was defined as follows: (1) elevations macroscopically not visible or just visible; (2) confined to the cartilage; and (3) noncomplementarily distributed on the cartilage surfaces. Cartilage characterized by absence of such elevation was called *smooth*. Cartilage characterized by the presence of just visible elevation was called

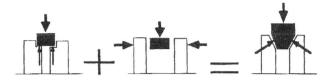

FIGURE 1.   The concepts of form closure (left), pure (theoretical) force closure (middle), and a combination of form and force closure (right).

coarse. Where a multitude of relatively large elevations was present, the coarseness was called *pronounced.* The features of the ridges and depressions were considered: (1) macroscopically clearly visible; (2) involving both cartilage and underlying bone; (3) complementary on both sides of the joint. Thus, adjoining surfaces were apt to fit snugly. The dissection specimens included a 12-year-old boy in whom the roughness in the joints was least but, nonetheless, distinctly present. In all other specimens a degree of roughness was observed; it was more prominent in adult men (Fig. 3). This dissection led to the conclusion that the observed roughening and increased coarseness of the auricular surfaces was a nonpathologic adaptation to the forces exerted on the sacroiliac joints leading to increased stability. It was noted parenthetically that the ridges and depressions can be mistaken roentgenographically for osteophytes.[4] Actual measurements of friction across these joints revealed a high coefficient.[33]

Movement and Governance of the Sacroiliac Articulation

In the first century B.C., Hippocrates recognized some movement of the sacroiliac joint in parturition but regarded it as immobile otherwise.[14] In the 17th century, Diemerbroch raised the suggestion that the articulation has some movement even in nonpregnant individuals.[3] The joint was categorized as a diarthrosis in 1864 by Von Luschka. The first supposition of a fixed axis of rotation came from research at the turn of the century. A recognition that buttock and leg pain may arise from hypermobility of the joint was raised by Goldthwait and Osgood[9] in 1905. Movement

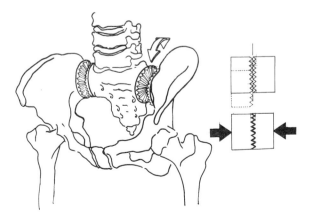

FIGURE 2.   The concept of stability at the sacroiliac articulation through the adducting effect of force closure and the concept of entrapment of one ilium in a more or less forward position are demonstrated.

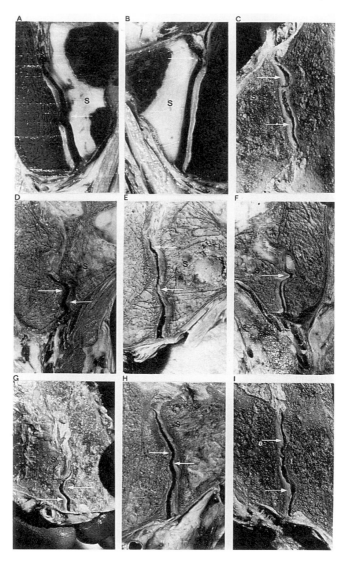

FIGURE 3. Frontal sections of the sacroiliac joints of embalmed specimens from males. S indicates the sacral side of the SI joint. *A* and *B* are from a 12-year-old boy. *C–I* are specimens from men older than 60. Arrows are directed at ridges and depressions. The ridges and depressions shown are covered by intact cartilage, which was checked by opening the joints afterward.

of these joints was accepted since then, although interest in the causes of pain in the buttock and leg was diverted to the complications of disk injuries by Mixter and Barr[15] in 1934. Despite a number of specific studies, interest in the movement of this joint has waned. Since 1954, and based on Weisl's work, the presence of some movement normally in the joint has become received opinion.[35] Nonetheless, many clinicians still hole that mobility is absent in the sacroiliac joints in adults (outside of the pregnant state) or is so slight that it is immaterial. Movement in living humans has been demonstrated stereophotogrammetically[25] with radiology by the placement of Kirschner wires in sacrum and ilium[2] and observing the external movement, and through actual measurements of iliac positions with calipers.[12,18] Motion at the sacroiliac joints is maintained even in advanced age.[34] Movement of these joints has been recognized in manual medical circles through methods of palpation throughout the history of osteopathy[10] and well established in physiotherapy circles as well.[5,11] Range of movement at the sacroiliac joint is indeed normally slight, and varying degrees of stiffness are present.

Governance of the joint is seemingly very little by way of the joint capsule itself, but mainly through the tightening of the several periarticular ligaments (see below). The capsule of the sacroiliac joint is frequently incomplete, as has been shown radiologically.[1] An analysis of movement at either sacroiliac articulation calls into question movement at the other two joints of the pelvic ring. Although interconnected through the soft tissues, the relative movement of each of the bones versus the others in the three directions of space, let alone the interaction with the fascial tube of the whole organism, creates a three-dimensional puzzle of great complexity. The osteopathic profession has labored with the classification of the *dysfunctions* of the axial skeleton for more than a hundred years. A recent classification[10] has brought some order into a subject that was previously marred with terminological turmoil. A reproducible, practical and uniformly applicable form of measurement of the relative movements of the four elements (fascia, sacrum, left ilium, and right ilium) has not been found. Manual palpation has not yielded interobserver consistency in measurements that are satisfactory for statistical analysis. Therefore, it remains only an impression of manual medical therapists that these movements can be palpated and treated.

A recent substantial meta-analysis of the cumulative research regarding the potential benefit of manual means of correcting back pain has confirmed its clinical benefit. However, the exact mechanism of action of manipulation remains speculative.

What can be said regarding the attendant ligaments and other soft tissue structures surrounding this joint? Research has shown that the large ligamentous bands, recognized of old in the pelvis, play substantial roles in the governance of the sacrum. Finally, to the extent that there is a *modal*—most typical pattern of movement round an hypothetical "axis"—it turns out that the deep posterior interosseous ligament of the sacroiliac joint plays that role.[8,25]

FUNCTION OF LIGAMENTS AND MUSCLE

Specific Ligaments

Nutation winds up the dense interosseous ligament of the sacroiliac joint, tightening and approximating the auricular surfaces, inducing the phenomenon of force closure. The important, and hitherto neglected, long dorsal sacroiliac ligament is, however, relaxed in nutation and tensed in counternutation.[28] This has been demonstrated in a recent study of 12 cadaver specimen performed at Erasmus University in Rotterdam, where tension was measured with a buckle transducer. In many patients with seemingly nonspecific low back pain, particularly in the peripartum period, the long posterior sacroiliac ligament is the source. Patients localize the pain to this site, which is also tender. This ligament is easily palpated just below the posterior superior iliac spine. (In our experience, this observation is true even in cases of arthrodesis of the sacroiliac articulations). Several structures, including the erector spinae muscle, the posterior layer of the thoracolumbar fascia, the sacrotuberous ligament,

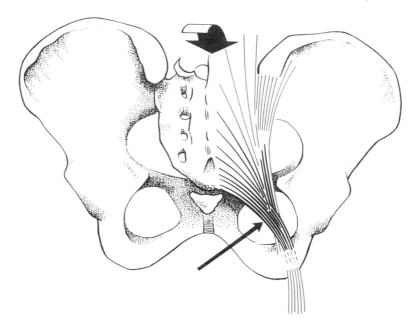

FIGURE 4. Tension in the body is transferred through ligaments and fasciae. The tendon of biceps femoris is seen here as continuous with the sacrotuberous ligament with a long posterior sacroiliac ligament and with the fascia over erector spinae. The long posterior sacroiliac ligament is relaxed in nutation.

and the sacrum, were incrementally loaded with forces up to 50 N. Forced nutation of the sacrum diminished the tension, and forced counternutation increased the tension of the long dorsal sacroiliac ligament. Tension also was increased during loading of the ipsilateral sacrotuberous ligament and erector spinae muscle. The tension decreased during traction of the gluteus maximus muscle and also with traction on the ipsilateral and contralateral posterior layer of the thoracolumbar fasciae in a direction simulating contraction of the latissimus dorsi muscle.[28] Slacking of the long dorsal sacroiliac ligament can be counterbalanced by both the sacrotuberous ligament and the erector spinae muscle.

Accordingly, clinicians need to keep in mind that pain localized within the boundaries of the long dorsal sacroiliac ligament might represent a spinal condition of sustained counternutation of the sacrum. In contrast, the sacrotuberous ligament is tightened in nutation.[30] This ligament functions as an extension of biceps femoris, assisting in the governance of the self-locking of the pelvis. This is how contraction of biceps femoris pulls on the soft tissues at the sacral side of the sacroiliac joint, thereby governing nutation (Figs. 4 and 5). The gluteus maximus, with its broad origin from the posterior and lateral aspect of the sacrum and sacrotuberous ligament below, as well as the fasciae above, is inserted predominantly into the greater trochanter of the femur. Its fascial origin is partly contiguous with the thoracolumbar fascia. It transfers force across the midline in the posterior layer of the thoracolumbar fascia, which is also tensioned by the contralateral latissimus dorsi.[29] Increased tension of the sacrotuberous ligament will preclude normal nutation of the sacroiliac joint.

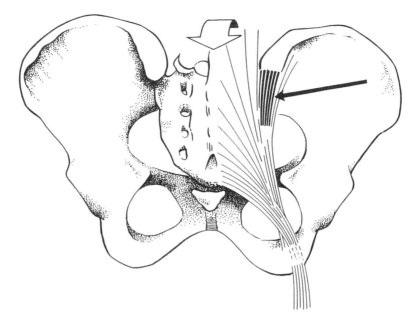

FIGURE 5. In counternutation, tension of the long posterior sacroiliac liagment is increased.

Muscle Function

Judging by their attachments, various muscles are probably involved, directly or indirectly, in force closure of the sacroiliac joints. The indirect effect is by *modulation of the tension* of ligaments and fascia. Each of these muscles have a somewhat variable "function," depending on the position of the two sacroiliac joints. These articulations are braced in nutation on stance, a situation that alternates between the sides in optimal healthy function. The sacroiliac articulations tend to be braced at most times. The degree of nutation/counternutation, interacting with the tension of the soft tissues around them, is variable. It affects, and is altered by, muscle action. The demarcation between normal and pathologic (positioning) is inconstant and has led to some terminological confusion. The common tendency for the articulation to drift into the suboptimal chronic position of an "anterior ilium" (i.e., a counternutated position) on one or both sides has been classified clinically[5] as pathologic, but an objective confirmation is still unavailable (see chapter 11). Four muscles will be analyzed as examples of modulators of fascial tension:

1. The erector spinae through its extending effect on the spine and its substantial sacral attachments might be expected to promote nutation. Since the muscle is a summation of many intersegmental units (catalogued under one name), it is likely that facilitation of select subsegments of this group of motorneurons might fire independently in certain situations. This is one of the many instances in which it is difficult to ascribe a prime movement to a trunk muscle because of the integrated function of the whole trunk.

2. The gluteus maximus muscle is large in the biped upright human stance but is diminutive in monkeys, which are essentially quadruped.[13] Some of the horizontal fibers of the gluteus maximus might be expected, on contraction, to have a direct

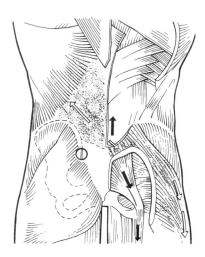

FIGURE 6. Diagrammatic representation of the major fascial layers of the low back. The right side shows (dark arrows) a part of the longitudinal muscle-tendon-fascia sling. Below, the continuation between the biceps femoris tendon and the sacrotuberous ligament with the erector spinae, above, illustrates functioning in concert (part of the thoracolumbar fascia has been removed). The left side shows the sacroiliac articulation (circled), and the open arrows indicate the pull of the latissimus dorsi, the posterior portion of the oblique abdominal muscles' fasciae connected to the thoracolumbar fascia, and continues with the gluteus maximus of the other side.

compressive effect on the sacroiliac articulations. The fibers attached to the sacrotuberous ligament are more interesting (the terms *origin* and *insertion* are more confusing than helpful here). When these fibers contract and raise the tension of the sacrotuberous ligament, self-locking is promoted and nutation governed. This is another example where, in addition to the 'prime function' of the muscle, one must recognize its role in modulating the tension of ligaments and fasciae. The effect of increasing the tension in the sacrotuberous ligament on the sacrum is variable and depends on posture and the existing degree of nutation.

3. The latissimus dorsi muscle is linked across the midline through the dorsolumbar fascia to the gluteus maximus of the other side. They seem to function in concert in trunk rotation. The thoracolumbar fascia can be tensed by the erector spinae muscle.[29] A correlation between the developmental mass of the erector spinae and tension in the thoracolumbar fascia has been demonstrated. Some of the interactions are shown in Figure 6.

4. The biceps femoris is an example of a limb muscle acting on what has traditionally been called its origin, also as a tensor of a ligament. The biceps femoris has been shown experimentally to alter the tension of the sacrotuberous ligament. In some specimens the attachment to the ischium was minimal, demonstrating that the main function is one of integrated tension modulation on the soft tissues, thereby controlling the main clutch of the trunk, the sacroiliac articulations[36] with incidental contact via a "toggle," the ischium. The measured tension in the ligament was affected by the degree of nutation of the sacrum and position of the rest of the body, which by inference is thought to affect the resting tension of the fascial ligamentous "tube" of the trunk.

Do any muscles maintain a state of continuous contraction to maintain the state of force closure—bracing—of the sacroiliac articulations? From a biomechanical perspective, something akin to a spring is "needed" to maintain the loaded closure pressure. Therefore, it seemed paradoxical that the in unconstrained sitting and standing, EMG testing showed the gluteus maximus and biceps femoris to be silent.[21] It turns out that, in this form of standing, the internal oblique abdominal muscles are under continuous tension. Voluntary muscles tend to relax cyclically (when they don't fatigue, spasm and trigger points develop). Nature's solution emerged from an experiment designed to falsify the hypothesis of muscle contributions to self bracing. It was found that when the legs are crossed the internal oblique ab-

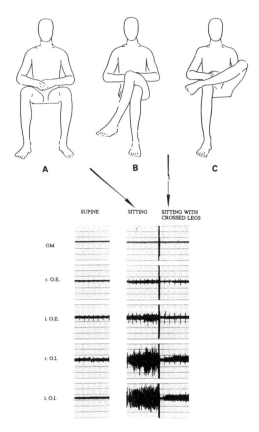

FIGURE 7. Sample electromyographic recordings are shown from supine, normal sitting, and cross-legged sitting. Decreased muscle activity, particularly that of the abdominal internal oblique muscles, in cross-legged sitting, can be seen. GM, gluteus maximus; OE, external oblique; OI, internal oblique; r and l indicate sides.

dominal muscles relax (Fig. 7). The trunk is rotated slightly, placing the fascial tube of the body under slight tension, which maintains compression of the pelvis. One ischium is subject to increased weightbearing, and the tensions measured in the latissimus dorsi of one side and the gluteus maximus of the other is increased. This balance can be maintained for some time, but creep in the soft tissue is apt to give enough slack after an interval, which will reflexly "wake up" the "guardian" internal obliques. At this point, a sitting person instinctively changes over to crossing the other leg.[22] It would be surprising if force closure were dependent on muscle action at rest, e.g., sitting. Therefore, the observation that adequate tension is generated in the fascia and ligaments to ensure force closure of the sacroiliac articulations by passive stretching—crossing the legs—is a reassuring and subtle instance of energy conservation.

Walking

We see, therefore, that the ligamentous and fascial surrounding structures (augmented by the large, flat musculature on both sides of the body) is importantly responsible for ipsilateral force closure of the sacroiliac articulation. The posterior layer of the thoracolumbar fascia acts as a large transmission belt. It is almost certain that, in walking, integrated action occurs between these several separately named anatomic entities. Additionally, if function of one component of this conglomerate is less than optimal, the role is taken over by the remaining functionally intact elements. Finally, even in cases in which the toggling synchronous alternating locking and release of one or other sacroiliac joint in stance or swing is impeded, walking can still take place because of the independent reserve function of the peripheral joints and muscles. It is proposed here that a complex interaction exists between all these elements in stance and swing, including (1) storage and release of elastic and (2) antigravitational energy,[6,7] (3) interactive complex motion of the compression and tension members of the pelvis, (4) and the surrounding ligaments and fasciae. The momentum in walking is a uniquely human physiologic process predicated on the peculiar anatomy of the sacroiliac articulations. The joint can be thought of as a multidirectional force transducer integrating the several functions of the pelvis discussed herein. Since the transducer involves an induction of energy and forces,[23] we suggest that this new concept of integrated function be called *transduction*. Transduction is defined as force closure alternating with the movement at the sacroiliac articulation in early swing (i.e., the integrated transfer of forces through the pelvis in stride) combined with the interactive normal motion of the sacrum the ilia and the lumbar spine in locomotion. Transduction is the process of the transfer of both elastic and gravitational forces between the pelvic components in kinetic motion.

CONCLUSION

The pelvis is central both anatomically and functionally in the human frame, which can be analyzed as a walking machine. This chapter has brought together evidence for a new understanding of the role of the sacroiliac joint as the key element in the pelvis. It allows the "walking machine" to transfer forces back and forth between the components of this "machine". Stance is afforded through force closure, which ensures stability. The joint allows the transfer and modulation of forces on the swing side. The integrated function of the whole pelvis facilitates efficient alternation of self-locking and energy transfer between the sides with each step. To comprehend this chapter, a number of new concepts are required:

- Force closure is a new concept that defines the clutch like bracing of a link in the closed kinematic chain of stance through friction—a function peculiar to human sacroiliac joints. It differs from form closure.
- Effective self-locking of the sacroiliac articulation is achieved through both form and force closure. Nutation winds up most of the ligaments in the area. Without nutation, effective self-locking would not occur. A "flexed" (or non-loaded) spine increases counter-nutation, tending to destabilize the pelvis.
- Locomotion transfers antigravitational and elastic energy back and forth between the moving parts. This is an essential function in walking because of the need to step.
- The ligaments around the joint play an essential role in its function. These roles include storage and release of elastic energy. An additional role is participation in the diffuse transfer of tension forces through the thoraco-lumbar fascia and, by analogy, through other fascial layers.
- The role of all the muscles in the trunk and lower limb is contributory, mostly as modulators of tension in the ligaments and fascia. The integrated function of these elements and forces is a characteristic of the human pelvis, ideally adapted to walking. This integrated function is called transduction.

REFERENCES

1. Aprill CN: The role of anatomically specific injections into the sacroiliac joint. First Interdisciplinary World Congress on Low Back Pain and its Relation to the Sacroiliac Joint, San Diego, November 1992. Rotterdam, ECO, 1992.
2. Colachis SC, Worden RE, Bechtol CO, et al: Movement of the sacro-iliac joint in the adult male: A preliminary report. Arch Phys Med Rehabil 44:490–498, 1963.
3. Diemerbroch I: The Anatomy of Human Bodies. (W. Salmon, trans). London, Brewster, 1689.
4. Dijkstra PF, Vleeming A, Stoeckart R: Complex motion tomography of the sacroiliac joint: An anatomical and roentgenological study. First Interdisciplinary World Congress on Low Back Pain and its Relation to the Sacroiliac Joint, San Diego, November 1992. Rotterdam, ECO, 1992, pp 301–309.
5. DonTigny RL: Mechanics and treatment of the sacroiliac joint. J Man Manip Ther 1:3–12, 1993.
6. Dorman T: Storage and release of elastic energy in the pelvis: Dysfunction, diagnosis, and treatment. J Orthop Med 14:54–62,1992.
7. Dorman TA, Cohen RE, Dasig D, et al: Energy efficiency during human walking; before and after prolotherapy. J Orthop Med 17:24–26, 1995.
8. Egund N, Olson TH, Schmid H, Selvik G: Movement in the sacroiliac joints demonstrated with Roentgen stereophotogrammetry. Acta Radiol Diag 19:833–846, 1978.
9. Goldthwait JE, Osgood RB: Essentials of body mechanics in health and disease.Med Surg J 152:593–634, 1905.
10. Greenman PE: Principles of Manual Medicine. Baltimore, Williams & Wilkins, 1989.
11. Hesch J: The Hesch Method of Treating Sacroiliac Joint Dysfunction. Albuquerque, J. Hesch, 1994.
12. LaCourse M, Moore K, Davis K, et al: A report on the asymmetry of iliac inclination: A study comparing normal, laterality and change in a patient population with painful sacro-iliac dysfunction treated with prolotherapy. J Orthop Med 12:69–72 1990.
13. Lovejoy CO: Evolution of human walking. Sci Am 82–89, 1988.
14. Lynch FW: Hippocrates according to Lynch: The pelvic articulations during pregnancy, labour and puerperium: An xray study. Surg Gynecol Obstet 300:357–580, 1920.
15. McDonald JA: Fibronectin: Extracellular Matrix Production and Remodeling. In Clark RAF, Henson PM (eds): The Molecular and Cellular Biology of Wound Repair. New York, Plenum Press, 1988 pp 405–436.
16. Mixter WJ, Barr JS: Rupture of intervertebral disc with involvement of spinal canal. N Engl J Med 211:210–215, 1934.
17. Popper KR: The Logic of Scientific Discovery. Harper & Row, 1959 (Translation of original German text, 1934).
18. Pitkin HC, Pheasant H: Sacrarthrogenic telalgia. A study of sacral mobility. J Bone Joint Surg 18: 365–374, 1936.
19. Russell ES: Form and Function: A Contribution to the History of Animal Morphology. Chicago, University of Chicago Press, 1982 (original, 1916).
20. Schekelle PG, Adams AH, Chassin MR, et al: The Appropriateness of Spinal Manipulation for Low-Back Pain. Santa Monica, CA, Rand, 1991.
21. Snijders CJ, Bakker MP, Vleeming A, et al: Oblique abdominal muscle activity in standing and in sitting on hard and soft seats. Clin Biomech 10:73–78, 1995.
22. Snijders CJ, Slagter AHE, van Strik R, et al: Why leg crossing? The influence of common postures on abdominal muscle activity. Spine 20:1995.
23. Snijders CJ, Vleeming A, Stoeckart R: Transfer of lumbosacral load to iliac bones and legs. Part 1: Biomechanics of self bracing of the sacroiliac joints and its significance for treatment and exercise. Clin Biomech 8:285–294, 1993.
24. Snijders CJ, Vleeming A, Stoeckart R: Transfer of lumbosacral load to iliac bones and legs. Part 2: Loading of the sacroiliac joints when lifting in a stooped posture. J Clin Biomech 8:295–301, 1993.
25. Sturesson B, Selvik G, Udèn A. Movement of the sacroiliac joints: A Roentgen stereophotogrammetic analysis. Spine 14:162–165, 1989.
26. Thompson DW: On Growth and Form. Cambridge, England, Cambridge University Press, 1961 (original, 1917).
27. Vleeming A: The sacroiliac joint. A clinical-anatomical, biomechanical and radiological study. Erasmus University, Rotterdam, 1990.
28. Vleeming A, Pool-Goudzwaard AL, Hammudoghlu D, et al: The function of the long dorsal sacroiliac ligament: Its implication for understanding low back pain. Spine (submitted).
29. Vleeming A, Pool-Goudzwaard AL, Stoeckart R, et al: The posterior layer of the thoracolumbar fascia; its function in load transfer from spine to legs. Spine (in press).

30. Vleeming A, Stoeckart R, Snijders CJ: The sacrotuberous ligament: A conceptual approach to its dynamic role in stabilizing the sacroiliac joint. Clin Biomech 4:201–203, 1989.

31. Vleeming A, Stoeckart R, Volkers ACW, Snijders CJ: Relation between form and function in the sacro-iliac joint. Part 1. Clinical-anatomical aspects. Spine 15:130–132, 1990.

33. Vleeming, A, Stoeckart, R, Volkers ACW, Snijders CJ: Relation between form and function in the sacro-iliac joint. Part 2. First Interdisciplinary World Congress on Low Back Pain and Its Relation to the Sacroiliac Joint. San Diego, November 1992. Rotterdam, ECO, 1992.

34. Vleeming A, Van Wingerden JP, Dijkstra PF, et al: Mobility in the sacroiliac joints in the elderly: A kinematic and radiologic study. Clin Biomech 7:170–176, 1992.

35. Weisl H: The relation of movement to structure in the sacro-iliac joint [doctoral thesis]. Manchester, England, University of Manchester, 1953.

36. Wingerden JP van, Vleeming A, Snijders CJ, Stoeckart R. A functional-anatomical approach to the spine-pelvis mechanism: Interaction between the biceps femoris muscle and the sacrotuberous ligament. Eur Spine I 2:140–144, 1993.

37. Wolff J: Die innere Architektur der Knochen. Arch Anat Phys 50: 1870.

C. J. SNIJDERS, PhD
A. VLEEMING, PhD
R. STOECKART, PhD
J. M. A. MENS, MD
G. J. KLEINRENSINK, MSc

BIOMECHANICAL MODELING OF SACROILIAC JOINT STABILITY IN DIFFERENT POSTURES

From the Department of
  Biomedical Physics and
  Technology (CJS)
Department of Anatomy (AV, RS,
  GJK)
Department of Rehabilitation
  Medicine (JMAM)
Erasmus University
Rotterdam
The Netherlands

Reprint requests to:
C. J. Snijders, PhD
Department of Biomedical Physics
  and Technology
Faculty of Medicine and Allied
  Health Sciences
P.O. Box 1738
3000 DR Rotterdam
The Netherlands

This chapter discusses the transfer of load from the spine to the innominate bones and legs, with special attention to the stability of the sacroiliac joints. Our interest in this topic was initiated by the earlier finding that in general the curvature of the lumbar spine in women is straighter before than after childbirth[19]; thus pain during pregnancy cannot be related to hollowing of the lumbar curvature. Because mechanical problems in the pelvis seemed to be a likely alternative cause, the logical step was the introduction in 1977 of a pelvic belt for treatment of peripartum pelvic pain; most patients reported a positive effect.[16] Although many factors may play a role, the belt was expected to have a direct mechanical effect on the stability of the sacroiliac joints. The following biomechanical model was developed by the Musculoskeletal Research Group, which consists of anatomists, physicists, engineers, and clinicians, in Rotterdam. The model begins with identification of the mechanical vulnerability of the sacroiliac joints. Mechanical solutions to protect the joints against dislocation are presented along with electromyographic and other findings that validate the underlying model.

BIOMECHANICAL MODEL

Mechanical Vulnerability of the Sacroiliac Joints

Maximal lumbosacral forces act on the vertebral column in a longitudinal direction, even in the

SPINE: State of the Art Reviews—Vol. 9, No. 2, May 1995
Philadelphia, Hanley & Belfus, Inc.

419

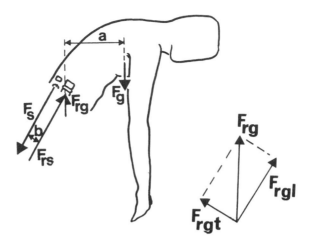

FIGURE 1.   Longitudinal forces on the spine ($F_{rs} + F_{rgl}$) are always greater than transverse forces (F_{rgt}), because the lever arm of the weight force (**a**) in stooped posture is greater than the lever arm of the counteracting dorsal muscles (**b**). (From Snijders CJ, Vleeming A, Stoeckart R: Transfer of lumbosacral load to iliac bones and legs. Part II: Loading of the sacroiliac joints when lifting in a stooped posture. Clin Biomech 8:295–301, 1993; with permission.)

forward-bending position (Fig. 1). The reaction force in the spine due to gravity (F_{rg}) has a transverse component (F_{rgt}) that is maximal when the trunk is in horizontal position and equals the weight of the upper body plus the weight in the hands. However, the longitudinal force on the spine is greater because of the unfavorable ratio between the lever arms of muscle force (F_s) and gravitational force (F_g) in relation to the intervertebral disks.[15] The position of the intervertebral disks is optimal, because they are perpendicular to the longitudinal orientation of the spine. However, the sacroiliac joint surfaces are parallel to the loading forces and are not protected

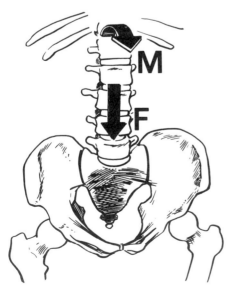

FIGURE 2.   Flat joints, such as the sacroiliac joints, are vulnerable to shear (rotation/translation) when loaded in the plane of the joint surfaces (M = moment, F = force). This observation leads to the hypothesis that compression of the joint surfaces by muscle force helps to prevent shearing.

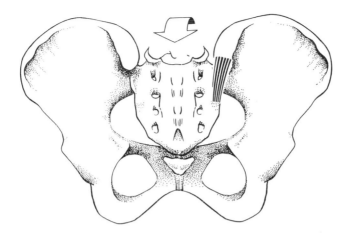

FIGURE 3. The long posterior sacroiliac ligament (right) connects the sacrum with the ilium and is tightened by counternutation (curved arrow). In this schematic drawing relations with other ligaments and fascia have been omitted.

against dislocation by the closed form of a ball-and-socket joint. Thus, the sacroiliac joints are vulnerable to shearing (translation, rotation) because of their predominantly flat surfaces,[17,23] which are almost parallel to the plane of maximal load (lumbosacral forces [F] and moments [M] in the sagittal plane) (Fig. 2).

A further assumption can be made with respect to resistance against nutation and counternutation of the sacrum. Vleeming et al.[25] point to the loading of the long dorsal sacroiliac ligament in counternutation (Fig. 3). This ligament was reported to be painful in 42% of patients with peripartum pelvic pain[9] and 44% with nonspecific low back pain.[11]

In lumbar kyphosis nutation is decreased. This so-called click-clack phenomenon[14] can be experienced when one sits upright on the edge of a straight chair. Slow forward translation of the trunk increases lumbar lordosis, whereas backward translation moves the center of gravity above the ischial tuberosities into an instable position. Further translation results in backward tilt of the pelvis and lumbar kyphosis. This transition from one stable position to another is called the lumbopelvic click-clack phenomenon (Fig. 4).

A further assumption is that, even when loading involves only the weight of the upper body, the sacroiliac joints are vulnerable to shearing as a consequence of liga-

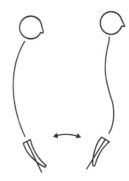

FIGURE 4. Translation of the trunk from a forward position to a backward position involves transition from one stable position to another in sitting. The intermediate posture with the center of gravity above the ischial tuberosities is an unstable position. This transition from lumbar lordosis to lumbar kyphosis is called the lumbopelvic click-clack phenomenon.

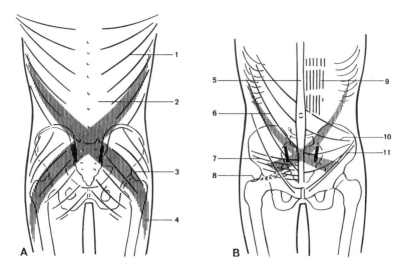

FIGURE 5. Trunk, arm, and leg muscles that compress the sacroiliac joints. The crosslike configuration indicates treatment and prevention of low back pain with strengthening and co-ordination of trunk, arm, and leg muscles in torsion and extension rather than flexion. *A,* latissimus dorsi (1), thoracolumbar fascia (2), gluteus maximus (3), iliotibial tract (4). *B,* linea alba (5), external abdominal obliques (6), transverse abdominals (7), piriformis (8), rectus abdominis (9), internal abdominal obliques (10), ilioinguinal ligament (11).

ment creep. Such deformation of the sacroiliac joints has been demonstrated in vitro.[24] Although the deformation is small, it promotes dislocation of the joints. Viscoelastic behavior also occurs in intervertebral disks,[5] but minor diminution in the height of the intervertebral disks does not imply dislocation of the joint.

Protection Against Shearing of Sacroiliac Joint Surfaces

Reports in the literature[2,6] assume that ligament structures ensure stability of the sacroiliac joints and that muscle forces are of no significance. In contrast, we assume that the ligament structures surrounding the sacroiliac joints are not capable of transferring lumbosacral load to the iliac bones in heavy-loading situations or in conditions with less but prolonged load (creep), such as standing and sitting. According to our model, resistance against shearing results from compression of the sacroiliac joint surfaces, which typically have a coarse texture, symmetric ridges and grooves, and an undulated shape. Compression can be produced by muscle forces, in combination with forces in ligaments and fascia, that cross the sacroiliac joint surfaces. This protective system requires the concerted action of muscles in the back, pelvis, and legs. Muscles with the appropriate direction are indicated in Figure 5.

The transverse section in Figure 6 shows how oblique abdominal muscle force compresses the sacroiliac joints. Because of the different lever arms of the abdominal muscle force and the force in the dorsal sacroiliac ligaments in relation to the sacroiliac joints, the magnification of the abdominal force resembles the mechanism of a nutcracker. Optimal function is obtained with stiff interosseous sacroiliac ligaments. Data from Miller et al.[10] indicate that this requirement is met.

A transverse section of the trunk distal to the umbilicus depicts the relationship between the internal abdominal oblique muscles and the thoracolumbar fascia (Fig. 7).

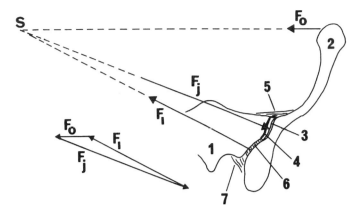

FIGURE 6. Cross-section of the pelvis at the level of the sacroiliac joints. Force application by the oblique abdominal muscles (F_o), in combination with stiff dorsal sacroiliac ligaments (F_l), compresses the sacroiliac joints (F_j). Because the lever arms of muscle and ligament force are different, the joint reaction force is much greater than the muscle force. Sacrum (1), iliac bone (2), joint cartilage (3), joint space (4), ventral sacroiliac ligament (5), interosseous sacroiliac ligaments (6), dorsal sacroiliac ligaments (7).

All forces raised by muscles in this cross-section create a reaction force in the spinal column and thus load the sacroiliac joints as well. Sacroiliac joint surfaces can also be protected against shearing by a loading mode that avoids shear. This interesting mechanical solution is created by the architecture of the pelvis, which resembles a Roman arch. The arch of the foot also illustrates this mechanism (Fig. 8).

The predominantly flat joint surfaces are loaded only with compression; shear is avoided.[17] The arch mechanism relies on the firm connection between the two

FIGURE 7. Cross-section of the trunk distal to the umbilicus with back muscles, deep lateral muscles, and abdominal muscles. Latissimus dorsi (1), erector spinae (2), the deep layer of the thoracolumbar fascia (3), the superficial layer of the thoracolumbar fascia (4), quadratus lumborum (5), psoas major (6), the body of the lumbar vertebra (7), linea alba (8), rectus abdominis (9), transverse abdominals (10), internal abdominal obliques (11), external abdominal obliques (12).

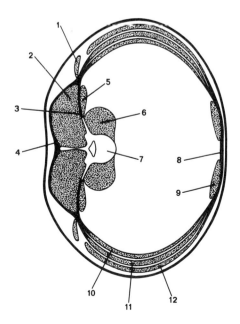

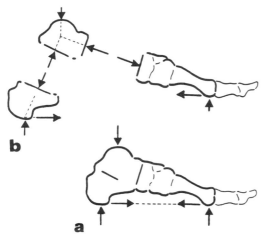

FIGURE 8. *A*, the arch of the foot compared with a Roman arch. *B*, flat joint surfaces in an arch experience compression while shear is avoided. (From Snijders CJ, Vleeming A, Stoeckart R: Transfer of lumbosacral load to iliac bones and legs. Part I: Biomechanics of self-bracing of the sacroiliac joints and its significance for treatment and exercise. Clin Biomech 8:285–294, 1993; with permission.)

ends. In the foot this function is ascribed to the plantar aponeurosis (among other structures), whereas in the pelvis such action can be ascribed to the sacrotuberous and sacrospinal ligaments, as well as the coccygeus and piriformis muscles. Figure 9 compares the arch of the foot and the arch of the pelvis. The effect of a pelvic belt distal to the sacroiliac joints can be seen as well. The pelvic arch receives bilateral support from the hip joints. When one sits on the ischial tuberosities, the supportive forces are below the sacroiliac joints and the mechanism of the arch is absent.

Erector Spinae Activity as a Support for Nutation

Movement of the sacrum into counternutation may be opposed by tension in the erector spinae muscles. However, this mechanism applies with certainty only to dorsal muscle force that acts on the sacrum (F_m) (Fig. 10). In combination with its reaction force (F_{rm}) in the spine F_m produces a couple-force that acts as a flexion

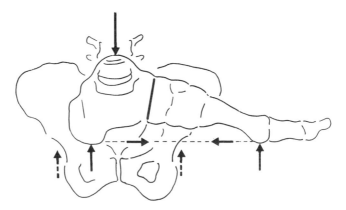

FIGURE 9. Analogy between the load on the sacroiliac joint and the load on a tarsal joint. The (horizontal) line of action of a pelvic belt distal to the sacroiliac joints is also seen. (From Snijders CJ, Vleeming A, Stoeckart R: Transfer of lumbosacral load to iliac bones and legs. Part I: Biomechanics of self-bracing of the sacroiliac joints and its significance for treatment and exercise. Clin Biomech 8:285–294, 1993; with permission.)

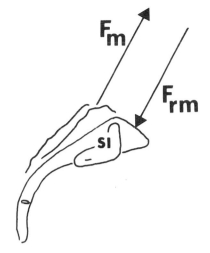

FIGURE 10. Parts of the erector spinae muscle are attached to the sacrum. Muscle force (F_m) and its reaction force in the spine (F_{rm}) form a couple-force that tends to move the sacrum into nutation. (From Snijders CJ, Vleeming A, Stoeckart R: Transfer of lumbosacral load to iliac bones and legs. Part II: Loading of the sacroiliac joints when lifting in a stooped posture. Clin Biomech 8:295–301, 1993; with permission.)

moment on the sacrum. Trunk muscles attached to the sacrum and trunk muscles attached to the iliac bones create a bifurcation in lumbosacral load.[18] Muscles attached to the iliac bones induce shear loading of the sacroiliac joints and possibly counter-nutation in certain postures.

VALIDATION OF THE BIOMECHANICAL MODEL

Biomechanical Studies

The concept of protection of the sacroiliac joints by muscle force agrees with reports that strenuous flexion-extension exercises and lifting[12,13] involve coordinated action of the hamstring, gluteus maximus, erector spinae, and latissimus dorsi muscles. Further validation was provided by electromyographic (EMG) studies of muscle activity in unconstrained postures. As expected, we found that in uncon-

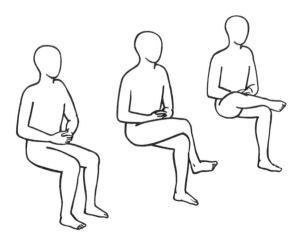

FIGURE 11. A, sitting on an office chair with a firm seat using backrest and armrests. B, upper legs crossed. C, ankle on knee. EMG recordings related to these postures are given in Figure 12.

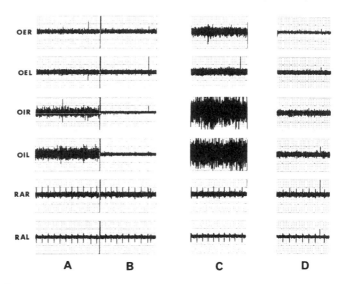

FIGURE 12. *A*, oblique abdominal muscles left (L) and right (R) are active in normal sitting. *B*, leg crossing leads to a significant decrease in internal oblique activity. *C*, oblique abdominal muscles are also active in unconstrained standing. Activity of erector spinae, gluteus maximus, and hamstring muscles, however, is absent. *D*, recording in supine position. OE = external oblique, OI = internal oblique, RA = rectus abdominus.

strained standing and in sitting with firm support of the trunk by a backrest, the activity of hamstring, erector spinae, and gluteus maximus muscles was low (comparable to levels in the supine position). If the biomechanical model of sacroiliac joint stability is correct, other muscles should act to compress the sacroiliac joints. Indeed, in both unconstrained standing and sitting the activity of oblique abdominal muscles was significant.

Because the continuous activity, especially of the internal oblique muscles, may be fatiguing, we looked for other mechanical solutions to stabilize the sacroiliac joints. Subjects sat on an office chair with a firm seat, backrest, and armrests. First we found that leg-crossing (upper legs crossed or ankle on knee) (Fig. 11) correlates with a significant decrease in activity of the internal obliques (Fig. 12).[21]

Another study focused on the pelvic arch. Geometry indicates that sitting on the ischial tuberosities will not stabilize the sacroiliac joints, which are located above the tuberosities. The model predicts, however, that lateral support restores the structure of the pelvic arch. Therefore we measured EMG activity of subjects sitting on the soft seat of an old car. Indeed, the decrease in internal oblique activity was considerable; levels were as low as in the supine posture[20] (Fig. 13).

The validation experiments also included loading tests on embalmed human specimens. Among other observations, we found that application of a pelvic belt increases the resistance of the sacroiliac joints to nutation and counternutation.[24]

Clinical Evidence

Since 1977 we have had positive experiences with the use of a pelvic belt in patients with peripartum pelvic pain.[16] Although this effect may be related to unknown factors (e.g., propriocepsis), we believe that the mechanical effect shown in vitro[24]

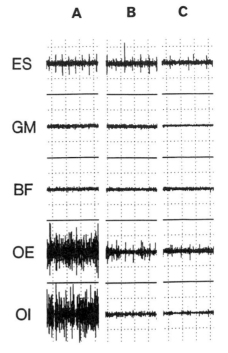

FIGURE 13. Unprocessed EMG signals recorded with the subject sitting on the hard seat of an office chair (*A*), sitting on a soft car seat (*B*), and supine (*C*). The difference in EMG activity on soft and hard seats is significant. ES = erector spinae, GM = gluteus maximus, BF = the long head of biceps femoris, OE = external oblique, OI = internal oblique. (From Snijders CJ, Bakker MP, Vleeming A, et al: Oblique abdominal muscle activity in standing and in sitting on hard and soft seats. Clin Biomech 10:73–78, 1995; with permission.)

also plays a role. The belt is often applied below the level of the sacroiliac joints, at the level of the greater trochanters. Other patients profit more from a belt just below the anterosuperior iliac spine or at the level of the pubic symphysis. Elastic pants also may be effective and often are more convenient. It is not necessary to pull the belt forcefully. Forces of approximately 50 N are sufficient (Fig. 14). However, if after 15 minutes no effect is observed the belt must not be pulled tighter; another so-

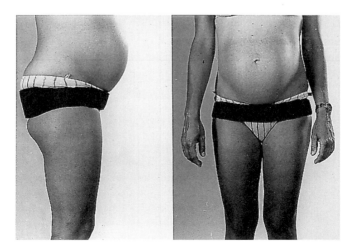

FIGURE 14. Often a pelvic belt reduces pain in the lower back and pelvis during pregnancy and after childbirth. A small force is sufficient.

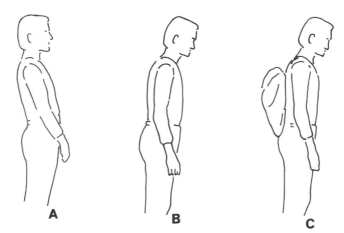

FIGURE 15. *A*, in erect posture iliopsoas muscles are always active, whereas erector spinae activity is absent. *B*, patients with low back pain often adopt a slightly stooped posture. Absence of iliopsoas activity means less load on the sacroiliac joints, whereas gravity load and erector spinae activity tend to move the sacrum into nutation, which is assumed to be favorable. *C*, application of a small rucksack diminishes erector spinae activity and may unload painful dorsal structures at the lumbopelvic level. The favorable slightly stooped posture, however, can be maintained.

lution must be sought. Pelvic belts are also beneficial in nonpregnant women and in men.[16]

Instead of standing upright, patients with low back pain often adopt a slightly forward-bent position (Fig. 15B). This position supports nutation of the sacrum for two reasons: (1) the component of gravitational force that acts on the top of the sacrum in a transverse direction becomes larger, and (2) the erector spinae muscle (see Fig. 10) becomes significantly active in a slightly stooped posture.[20] Furthermore, this posture may relax the iliopsoas muscle and unload the sacroiliac joints, because the forces exerted by the vertebral portion of the psoas muscle on the sacrum run almost parallel to the sacroiliac joints. The psoas muscles are continuously active in erect postures,[1] and release of tension may correlate with reduction of lumbar lordosis.[14]

In the slightly forward-bent position, the erector spinae muscle may load painful structures—for instance, through its connection with the long dorsal sacroiliac ligaments.[25] In a pilot EMG study we demonstrated that the added weight of a small rucksack decreases erector spinae activity (Fig. 15C). Although this test involved subjects without low back pain, the results may explain the resolution of pain and the improved mobility after application of a small rucksack (3 kg) in the treatment of peripartum pelvic pain (J.M.A. Mens, unpublished data). Similar effects were observed in male patients with low back pain. Although such observations are promising, they remain preliminary.

Physicians can simulate the action of a pelvic belt as well as of the oblique abdominal muscles (see Fig. 6) by applying medially directed manual forces to one or both hip bones. Patients with peripartum pelvic pain and instability severe enough to inhibit lifting their legs while lying supine found that this function could be restored by a manually applied adducting force across the pelvis through the iliac bones. The

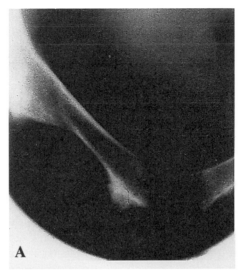

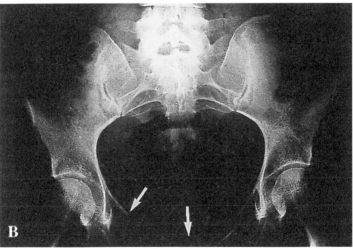

FIGURE 16. Radiographs of a 34-year-old woman before (*A*) and after (*B*) resection (arrows) of the pubic bone because of a chondrosarcoma. Mechanical function remained normal. (From Snijders CJ, Vleeming A, Stoeckart R: Transfer of lumbosacral load to iliac bones and legs. Part I: Biomechanics of self-bracing of the sacroiliac joints and its significance for treatment and exercise. Clin Biomech 8:285–294, 1993; with permission.)

applied force is approximately 50 N. This clinical test may be interpreted as a strong validation experiment for the biomechanical model of the sacroiliac joints. Some weight lifters use a special belt that is dorsally wide but narrow at the ventral side. Such belts are applied forcefully around the cranial side of the iliac crest. The mechanism of action is ascribed to an increase in intraabdominal pressure, which gives extra support to the back. Magnetic resonance imaging (MRI) showed that such belts act at the level of the sacroiliac joints,[18] and we hypothesized that the belt contributes to stability of the sacroiliac joints in a stooped posture.

In the biomechanical model on sacroiliac joint stability[17] the symphysis has no role. Thus the concept of the "pelvic ring" is not required for the modeling of transfer of large lumbosacral loads to the legs. Supporting evidence may be found in the radiographs (Fig. 16) of a 34-year-old woman with chondrosarcoma, before and after resection of the pubic bone. In a follow-up period of 4 years the mechanical function remained normal, with no complaints from the patient. Symphysiolysis may be associated with hypermobility of the sacroiliac joints. Therefore, isolated surgical symphysiodesis can be questioned; it interferes with proper function of sacroiliac load transfer and does not resolve the problem of sacroiliac joint instability.

DISCUSSION AND CONCLUSIONS

The starting point for the biomechanical model of the sacroiliac joints is their vulnerability during transfer of lumbosacral load to the iliac bones and legs, including large loads in stooped postures as well as moderate loads in unconstrained standing and sitting. In asymmetric postures, such as the one-leg stance, transfer of lumbosacral load is concentrated on one sacroiliac joint. Thus lifting with torsion of the trunk involves risk of injury, because it is associated with unequal distribution of the load on the legs.

Based on clinical evidence and biomechanical tests, it is assumed that overload of dorsal sacroiliac ligaments may result from forcing the sacrum into counternutation. Such forcing may be related to an abrupt transition from lumbar lordosis to lumbar kyphosis, which we have called the lumbopelvic click-clack phenomenon. Because of the analogy with a sprained ankle, we are especially interested in "sprain of the lower back." Similarities include severe pain, which usually resolves spontaneously; strong muscle tension, which initially resists movement; and swelling with possible nerve entrapment. In both cases the treatment of choice is to keep the patient moving. Ankle strain occurs in one direction (i.e., inversion trauma), which may be compared with counternutation of the sacrum (i.e., retroflexion trauma).

Because our biomechanical model of sacroiliac joint stability depends on muscle activity, protection against retroflexion trauma depends on the rate of muscle action; the muscle forces must be generated at precisely the right time. This process may be viewed as "joint protecting" or "arthrokinetic" reflex.[4] Impairment of elements in reflex chains may cause delayed muscle reaction and impair the functional stability of joints. This instability may be of short duration (the velocity of load application is once-only greater than the reaction time of the muscles) or become chronic. A permanent injury of one of the elements of the reflex chain may involve a permanent discrepancy between the velocity of load application and the reaction time of the muscles. Kleinrensink et al.[7] showed a relation between inversion trauma and impaired function of the peroneal nerve, which transmits both afferent and efferent information in the arthrokinetic reflex chain of the ankle. This relation may explain recurrences.

Craniocaudal reflexes due to flexion or extension of the head also may play a role in loading and stability of the sacroiliac joints.

In addition to abrupt forcing, overload of dorsal sacroiliac ligaments also may be related to lower but prolonged load, as in sitting with lumbar kyphosis caused by lack of a proper backrest.

The integrity of the sacroiliac joints depends on a strong ligamentous system. The present study, however, focuses on whether additional mechanical provisions contribute to sacroiliac joint stability. Several mechanical solutions depend on geometry. The main conclusion is that muscle forces are needed in almost all modes of sacroiliac load; exceptions were found during the validation experiments. During unconstrained sitting with the support of a backrest and armrests the activity in the oblique abdominal muscles appeared to decrease significantly when subjects crossed their legs or when they sat on a soft car seat.

The model points to specific muscles that, in combination with ligaments and fascia, produce forces that cross the sacroiliac joints and increase compression of the joint surfaces, resulting in resistance to shearing. Muscles that act in the sagittal plane (parallel to the sacroiliac joint surfaces) are expected to produce unfavorable forces (e.g., the rectus abdominis and the vertebral part of the iliopsoas). Thus treatment and prevention of low back pain should be based on strengthening and coordination of trunk, arm, and leg muscles in torsion and extension rather than flexion.

The biomechanical model helps to understand positive experiences with well-established treatment modalities. But it also leads to new ideas for diagnosis and treatment. For example, in patients with peripartum pelvic pain who cannot lift their legs in a supine posture, application of moderate force to the hip bones in a medial direction restores the ability to lift the legs.[8]

Because it is difficult to assess the mobility of the sacroiliac joints in an objective way, a new method was developed.[3] After validation experiments in embalmed human specimens, different degrees of stiffnesses could be identified in the sacroiliac joints of healthy subjects and patients. With subjects in a prone position, moderate vibrations were applied to the anterosuperior iliac spine in an anteroposterior direction. At the dorsal side the vibrations were imaged with color Doppler at both sides of the ipsilateral sacroiliac joint.

A new concept for treatment is application of a small rucksack to relieve pain and to improve mobility in patients with low back pain. Although the initial results are promising, further clinical experience is needed. However, the biomechanical model explains these and other observations.

ACKNOWLEDGMENTS

The authors thank G.A. Hoek van Dijke, M.T.L.M. Ribbers, R. Niesing, C. de Vries, and J.V. de Bakker for their valuable contributions.

REFERENCES
1. Basmajian FV, De Luca CJ: Muscles Alive: Their Functions Revealed by Electromyography. Baltimore, Williams & Wilkins, 1985.
2. Bernard TN Jr, Cassidy JD: The sacroiliac joint syndrome: Pathophysiology, diagnosis and treatment. In Vleeming A, Mooney V, Snijders CJ, Dorman T (eds): Proceedings of the First Interdisciplinary World Congress on Low Back Pain and its Relation to the Sacroiliac Joint. San Diego, 1992, pp 119–124.
3. Buyruk HM, Stam HJ, Snijders CJ, et al: Assessment of sacroiliac joint mobility by dynamic testing of a pelvis model [abstract]. Second World Congress of Biomechanics, July 10–15, 1994, Amsterdam. Vol. 1, p 269.
4. Cohen LA, Cohen ML: Arthrokinetic reflex of the knee. Am J Physiol 184:433–437, 1956.
5. Dieën JH van, Toussaint HM: Spinal shrinkage as a parameter of functional load. Spine 18:1504–1514, 1993.
6. Grieve EFJ: Mechanical dysfunction of the sacroiliac joint. Int Rehabil Med 5:46–52, 1983.
7. Kleinrensink GJ, Stoeckart R, Meulstee J, et al: Lowered motor conduction velocity of the peroneal nerve after inversion trauma. Med Sci Sports Exerc 26:877–883, 1994.
8. Mens JMA, Vleeming A, Snijders CJ, Stam HJ: A theoretical model of the pelvis and its clinical consequences: A study of patients with peripartum pelvic instability. In Proceedings of the Second Interdisciplinary World Congress on Low Back Pain. The Integrated Function of the Lumbar Spine and Sacroiliac Joints. San Diego, November 9–11, 1995.
9. Mens JMA, Stam HJ, Stoeckart R, et al: Peripartum pelvic pain: A report of the analysis of an inquiry among patients of a Dutch patient society. In Vleeming A, Mooney V, Snijders CJ, Dorman T

(eds): Proceedings of the First International Congress on Low Back Pain and Its Relation to the Sacroiliac Joint. San Diego, 1992, pp 119–144.

10. Miller JAA, Schultz AB, Andersson GBJ: Load-displacement behavior of sacroiliac joints. J Orthop Res 5:92–101, 1987.
11. Njoo KH: Regional pain syndromes in patients with low back pain. In preparation.
12. Noe DA, Mostardi RA, Jackson ME, et al: Myoelectric activity and sequencing of selected trunk muscles during isokinetic lifting. Spine 17:225–229, 1992.
13. Oddsson L, Thorstensson A: Fast voluntary trunk flexion movements in standing: Motor patterns. Acta Physiol Scand 129:93–106, 1987.
14. Snijders CJ: On the form of the human thoraco-lumbar spine and some aspects of its mechanical behaviour. Thesis, Eindhoven, 1970.
15. Snijders CJ, Nordin M, Frankel VH: Biomechanica van het spier-skeletstelsel; Grondslagen en toepassingen. Utrecht, Lemma, 1995.
16. Snijders CJ, Snijder JGN, Hoedt HTE: Biomechanische modellen in het bestek van rugklachten tijdens de zwangerschap. T Soc Gezondheidszorg 62:141–147, 1984.
17. Snijders CJ, Vleeming A, Stoeckart R: Transfer of lumbosacral load to iliac bones and legs. Part I: Biomechanics of self-bracing of the sacroiliac joints and its significance for treatment and exercise. Clin Biomech 8:285–294, 1993.
18. Snijders CJ, Vleeming A, Stoeckart R: Transfer of lumbosacral load to iliac bones and legs. Part II: Loading of the sacroiliac joints when lifting in a stooped posture. Clin Biomech 8:295–301, 1993.
19. Snijders CJ, Seroo JM, Snijder JGN, Hoedt HT: Change in form of the spine as a consequence of pregnancy. Ottawa, Digest 11th ICMBE, 1976, pp 670–671.
20. Snijders CJ, Bakker MP, Vleeming A, et al: Oblique abdominal muscle activity in standing and in sitting on hard and soft seats. Clin Biomech 10:73–78, 1995.
21. Snijders CJ, Slagter AHE, Strik R van, et al: Why leg-crossing? The influence of common postures on abdominal muscle activity. Spine 20: 1995.
22. Vleeming A, Stoeckart R, Volkers ACW, Snijders CJ: Relation between form and function in the sacroiliac joint. Part I: Clinical anatomical aspects. Spine 15:130–132, 1990.
23. Vleeming A, Volkers ACW, Snijders CJ, Stoeckart R: Relation between form and function in the sacroiliac joint. Part II: Biomechanical aspects. Spine 15:133–136, 1990.
24. Vleeming A, Buyruk HM, Stoeckart R, et al: An integrated therapy for peripartum pelvic instability: A study of the biomechanical effects of pelvic belts. Am J Obstet Gynecol 166:1243–1247, 1992.
25. Vleeming A, Pool-Goudzwaard AL, Hammudoghlu D, et al: The function of the long dorsal sacroiliac ligament: Its implication for understanding low back pain (submitted).

THOMAS A. DORMAN, MD

THE SLIPPING CLUTCH SYNDROME

Private Practice
San Luis Obispo, California

Look at a person standing and walking. The great sections of the organism are the trunk and the two legs. They are brought together at the pelvis, at the core of which is the sacrum, a trapezoid, wedge-shaped bone. As discussed in chapter 6, this bone, the core of the body, is located and buffeted by the forces around it. These are the forces of locomotion, walking being the prime function of the mechanics of the human upright body. The attachments of the sacrum to the rest of the soma are strong. The multiple ligaments maintain the sacrum's position between the ilia on the two sides, the fifth lumbar vertebra and the rest of the spinal column above, and the coccyx below. Virtually all of the fascial sheaths, the transmission belts of forces that convey the energy of locomotion back and forth among the trunk and each leg, are arrayed around it and transfer force about, but not through, the sacrum. Therefore, the sacrum acts as a passive wedge that is located centrally among these forces.

The role of its major attachments, the posterior sacroiliac ligaments, is that of springs. They store and release elastic energy with the cyclic torque of the ilia within the pelvic ring and about the approximate axis of nutation and counternutation. This axis is approximately through the deep interosseous ligaments. These ligaments do not lie in any of the primary geometric body planes but lie approximately diagonally, anteroposteriorly, mediolaterally, and superior to inferior from the medial to the lateral aspect. The interosseous (sometimes called innominate) core of the posterior sacroiliac ligaments are the thickest ligaments in humans and are extraordinarily short, consisting of fibers of collagen twisted around each other like a rope. Shortening occurs through this mechanism, with torque. This allows bracing of the auricular surfaces of the sacroiliac joint to each other, as discussed in chapters 9 and 10. With each step, the ilia toggle or rotate back and forth, the sacrum on the stance side being positioned in counternutation and on the swing side moving into nutation. The sacrum, versus the trunk as a whole, has an oscillating normal movement approximating a figure eight.

The ilia do not rest symmetrically about the sacrum within the pelvis. In fact, the right ilium is slightly forward in right-handed individuals, and the opposite is true in left-footed individuals.[2]

As discussed in chapter 9, stability in stance is maintained through self-bracing, also defined by Vleeming as force closure. It should be plain to the reader by now that self-bracing in stance is predicated on firm contact between the rough auricular surfaces of the sacroiliac articulations. The rope ties these articulations together, and the posterior sacroiliac iliac ligaments are controlled predominantly by the interosseous component. All other tension members traversing the trunk contribute indirectly to the tension mechanism called the pelvis and that has been defined as the tensegrity model (see chapters 5 and 7). The extraordinary feature of this mechanism is the passivity of the movement of the sacrum. The sacrum affords attachment to the origin of the piriformis muscle ventrally and to the multifidus muscle dorsally. They are prime movers of the sacrum. Nonetheless, the sacrum's main role—being wedged and affording stability and torque alternately between the sides in the process of locomotion—is essentially passive.

A Surprise

Viewed in this perspective, it should not be surprising that dysfunction of this passive, trapezoid, wedged keystone can occur when the ligaments relax and when an asymmetric pull occurs across any of the multiple fascial and ligamentous attachments of any of the soft tissues transferring forces across the core of the pelvis. This confirms the long-standing osteopathic tenet that somatic dysfunction in the pelvis is the rule and that correction of pelvic dysfunction is cardinal in restoration of optimal symmetry and usually contributes to the abolition of pain. This is the case whether the concentration of strain, the symptomatic pain, is at the pelvic girdle itself or elsewhere in the axial skeleton or elsewhere in the "fascial tube" we call our bodies. Referred pain and referred strains through this tensegrity mechanism are almost always associated with asymmetric entrapment of the sacrum between the ilia, that is, somatic dysfunction in the pelvis. As discussed in chapter 3, some degree of asymmetric entrapment is normal in the sense that it is statistically usual; when exaggerated, it amounts to disease, i.e., somatic dysfunction.

The reductionist evidence for these statements is presented throughout this volume. The reader will need to accept that the main thrust of the argument is the gestalt of osteopathy. Manual medicine achieves the same end whether practiced by osteopaths, chiropractors, physiotherapists, or even in antiquity by manipulators of the axial skeleton, and whether it is intentionally or by inchoate reasoning aimed at the sacroiliac articulations. Is it possible that these manual approaches are effete, a massive mistake, charlatanism, and wrong? Could the tradition of manipulation, with its multiple starts, dismissals, and recurrences have been one great accident? It would be rash to assume that so many common themes would have arisen merely by chance; the obvious conclusion is that manipulation of the pelvis has a basis in reality. Adherence to the dogma of immobility at the pelvic ring flies in the face of common sense. Would nature maintain a joint where no motion occurs? An authoritarian meta-analysis has established the role of manipulation in back pain, even if it has not defined the mode of action.[5]

Serendipity

Discoveries often occur from the coincidence of two observations. The discovery of the *slipping clutch syndrome* followed this pattern. This author had a number of patients with back pain—in whom dysfunction at the posterior sacroiliac ligaments was being treated by prolotherapy with Ongley's technique—who had the additional and, at first, seemingly unconnected occurrence of episodic falling. The main features of this phenomenon, now called slipping clutch syndrome, include a history of an injury, usually a fall before the onset of the two problems: (1) back pain, usually with radiation into one buttock and leg, and (2) episodic falling. Falling occurs irregularly and unexpectedly. This has been defined by John Mennell as an *intrinsic injury*.[3]

Contrast this with the accounts patients give of falling when an external circumstance is responsible, such as an unexpected step, a pothole, a slippery surface. In slipping clutch syndrome, the falls rise from an intrinsic cause. Patients recognize that the fault is *within* and are usually embarrassed. They generally do not connect the slipping clutch syndrome with their back pain. Since patients often fail to report their episodes of falling, clinicians should solicit the patient's account of a fall with specific questioning.

Since recognizing this syndrome, the author has systematically asked patients with back pain about episodes of falling and has elicited a higher incidence of this symptom than previously recognized. Now that inquiries about falling have become routine, a lesser degree of this phenomenon is coming to light: patients report a sense of giving way, as if the leg is about to fail to serve as a stable brace on stance, but "I am able to catch myself, Doctor." This characteristic is distinctly common in individuals with severe sacroiliac dysfunction—in this author's experience, about 15% of patients with back pain.

At first, this writer failed to associate episodic falling with the sacroiliac joint even though it was during this time that research about the role of the ligaments in the pelvis was just beginning. Then, patients who received treatment with prolotherapy to the posterior sacroiliac ligaments began to express gratitude that their episodic falling had been corrected. It was thereby through serendipity that the diagnosis of the slipping clutch syndrome was made. The cure for episodic falling clinched not only the treatment for episodic falling, but its actual mechanism was brought to light. Therefore, it is proposed here that the delicate balance of bracing on the stance side and release and swing on the swing side of the toggle mechanism, the sacrum, is where dysfunction can occur. The dysfunction can take three forms, as follows:

1. An enhanced degree of asymlocation (somatic dysfunction) associated with enhanced strain on one or other ligament. The strain will generate prolonged pain, which may be sensed over the ligament or be *referred*. From this arises the multitude of painful conditions in and around the pelvis.

2. The pelvic dysfunction will have secondary effects along the tensegrity model, or axial skeleton. The resulting strain probably will be present at remote sites, which are at risk of becoming pain generators in their own right.

3. If self-bracing fails momentarily at the first point of contact between the two rough auricular surfaces in stance and a slight degree of slippage occurs after the initiation stance, the person will lose balance at the critical moment of transfer-

ring weight onto the stance leg in the support phase. This minor shift will cause a loss of balance and falling or a sense of giving way with the person catching himself or herself before the fall is complete. Restoration of function at the interosseous ligaments and other parts of the posterior sacroiliac ligamentous system corrects all of these dysfunctions, including episodic slippage.

An article has been published describing the beneficial outcome of treatment with Ongley's technique, predominantly with prolotherapy to the aposterior sacroiliac articulations. Incidental correction of failure of self-bracing of the sacroiliac articulation occurred in all eight participants.[1]

SUMMARY

It was through serendipity that the treatment established for the recognized dysfunction of the posterior sacroiliac ligaments—pain and episodic displacement—also cured the third manifestation of the dysfunction, the dynamic one of the slipping clutch. Through recognition of the hitherto unexpected cure for the episodes of falling, the syndrome was described.

It is a subtle concept that association can be made between observations. In the presence of a theory, the association can be interpreted as confirming or denying a hypothesis.[4] Causation, however, is strictly in the mind of the scientist; causation itself is a philosophical concept. To that extent, one must accept Karl Popper's philosophical limitation: causation and scientific theories are merely temporary intellectual housings for associated phenomena. They can be thought of as a mental tool that allows us to associate phenomena, relate them intellectually, hold them together in our minds, and manipulate them for practical use. Any theory survives only until empiric observations deny its tenets. Copernican hypotheses have replaced the Ptolemaic, and Einsteinian relativity is still buffeting Gallilean and Newtonian mechanics.

This writer proposes that the best present hypothesis on the role of the human pelvis is that of a transducer for the transfer of forces for locomotion between the three main anatomic elements: the trunk and the two legs. Knowledge of form and function, anatomy and physiology, has allowed us to study dysfunction. In the case of the dysfunction of the human pelvis, this approach has yielded results just as beneficial as it has in other branches of biology and medicine. The scientist needs, however, to accept that in the context of dysfunction of the axial skeleton and the pelvis in particular, the concepts of asymlocation, entrapment, self-bracing, and force closure are necessary tools; from these, the recognition of the slipping clutch syndrome is a mere small step.

REFERENCES

1. Dorman T: Failure of self bracing at the sacroiliac joints: The slipping clutch syndrome. J Orthop Med 16:49–51,1994.
2. LaCourse M, Moore K, Davis K: A report on the asymmetry of iliac inclination: A study comparing normal, laterality and change in a patient population with painful sacro-iliac dysfunction treated with prolotherapy. J Orthop Med 12:69–72,1990.
3. Mennell J: Back Pain. Boston, Little, Brown & Co., 1960.
4. Popper KR: The Logic of Scientific Discovery. New York, Harper & Row, 1959 (Translation of original German text, 1934).
5. Shekelle PG, Adams AH, Chassin MR, et al: Spinal manipulation for low-back pain. Ann Intern Med 117:590–598, 1992.

THOMAS H. RAVIN, MD

IMAGING MECHANICAL DYSFUNCTIONS OF THE SPINE

From the Val d'Isere Health Clinic
Denver, Colorado

Reprint requests to:
Thomas H. Ravin, MD
45 South Dahlia
Denver, CO 80222

The documentation of mechanical dysfunctions by imaging techniques has challenged radiologists for a hundred years. In turn, the revival of manipulation as a spinal treatment option[28] challenges imagers to prove in black, white, and grays abnormalities that are palpable. State-of-the-art radiographic evaluation of mechanical dysfunction of the spine combines new ideas and techniques with those that are old and proven but nearly forgotten. The treatment of spinal pain with manipulation and injection therapies increases the importance of images in the assessment of minor congenital anomalies, mechanical dysfunction, and ligamentous laxity. The ability of radiologists to aid in the diagnosis and treatment of such problems has been lost in the specialization of medicine. Few radiologists can identify the simplest of somatic joint dysfunctions with their hands, and few clinicians can identify the presence of osteitis condenses illi on a plain film. This chapter hopes to bridge part of the gap.

Ferguson,[9] Fryette,[13] Mitchell,[27] and other clinicians of the 1930s and 1940s combined both clinical and imaging skills. Their observations of an unlevel sacral base,[4] lumbosacral joint orientation, and the lumbosacral angle have remained the standard for 50 years since they were first described. Their observations, combined with contemporary descriptions of spinal mechanics, allow images to become valuable aids to the treating clinician. The identification of congenital anomalies, pubic dysfunction, sacroiliac joint arthritis, and coccygeal displacements on radiographs elucidates the causes of the painful low back.

SPINE: State of the Art Reviews—Vol. 9, No. 2, May 1995
Philadelphia, Hanley & Belfus, Inc.

437

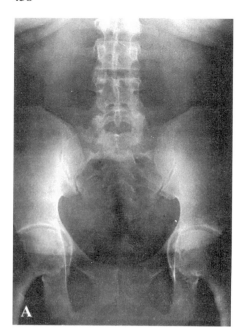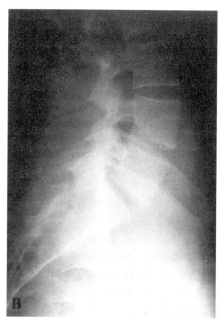

FIGURE 1. *A*, standing anteroposterior (AP) view of pelvis and lumbar spine. Note that the central beam of the x-ray is at L4. One should be able to visualize the symphysis pubis and the femoral heads as well as the lower lumbar spine. *B*, a lateral (Lat) pelvis and lumbar spine film also has the central beam at L4. Ideally the image should visualize the coccyx and the pubes.

The reawakening interest in the cervical spine and the painful sequelae of whiplash-associated disorders has created a renewed interest in imaging this area. Jackson's summation of radiographic findings in the cervical spine remain as pertinent today as 25 years ago.[20] In the cervical spine the presence of small but significant subluxations of vertebrae, uneven opening and closing of spinous processes in flexion and extension, and short-curve scoliosis are "tracks" of mechanical dysfunctions.

The evaluation of the spine with computer-aided images has opened new vistas for observations about mechanical dysfunctions.[11] When these images are added to plain x-ray films, considerable information about the functions of the spine is possible. Mechanical dysfunctions of the lower spine, such as rotated vertebrae and sacral twists, asymlocations, and even torsions or abnormal positions of the sacrum in several planes are present on many examinations of the spine. Their presence is seldom mentioned in radiographic reports.

TECHNIQUE

The radiographic techniques of low back imaging are generally well known but merit brief review. Most lumbosacral films should be taken with the patient standing. The basic examination consists of an anteroposterior film of the lumbar spine and pelvis and a lateral film of the lumbosacral spine. The feet are shoulder width apart, and the weight is equally distributed between the two legs. The importance of this positioning cannot be overstated; without weight-bearing films, the ability to communicate similar findings between physicians is lost. Anteroposterior films of the lumbar spine with the patient on a horizontal table are worthless from the functional point of view. Such films are good only for evaluating whether the patient has the proper number of bones and whether fractures are present. The main exception is measurement of Ferguson's angle (see below).

The film of the pelvis also should be taken so that the central ray of the beam (where the cross-hairs point) is at the L4 level. This technique reveals a good view of most of the structures of the lumbar spine and pelvis as well as a view of the femoral heads, coccyx, and symphysis pubis. Figure 1A is an example of a normal lumbar spine with the patient and film in good alignment. Note the position of the symphysis pubis and how the femoral heads are visualized. The patient is standing squarely between the edges of the film.

On the lateral spine film, the patient should be positioned with the central beam at L4 and centered nicely between the two edges of the film (Fig. 1B). In the lateral view the technique should be adjusted so that good detail of the lumbosacral junction, coccyx, and symphysis pubis can be well visualized. This requires an increase in the amount of radiation because of the thickness of the patient.

The cervical spine also should be imaged with the patient standing. Because of the loads of gravity, the cervical spine often demonstrates persistent changes that are not present when the patient is lying down. As in the lumbar spine, horizontal images should be reserved for the emergency department examination.

Functional imaging of the cervical and lumbar spines may include lateral flexion and extension films. In some cases these images define the nature of mechanical joint dysfunctions. The third set of films that occasionally may be obtained are oblique views for the evaluation of spondylolisthesis in the low back and size of the neural canals in the cervical spine.

CONGENITAL ABNORMALITIES AND MECHANICAL DYSFUNCTIONS

The relationship between congenital abnormalities and mechanical dysfunctions is perhaps the single most important reason to image the lumbar spine. The reported incidence of clinically significant congenital abnormalities ranges from 6%[14] to 50%.[9] In the 1930s, Ferguson, Fryette, and others began to notice the relationship between certain congenital abnormalities and low back pain. They observed that several common congenital anomalies, particularly those involving the lumbosacral joints, were frequently associated with low back pain. These radiographic observations and their clinical corollaries became separated over the years, but the issues have been periodically reunited.[8,19] In the twilight of the twentieth century, with a rising interest in nonsurgical care of the back, it is again time to read these gems of clinical imaging literature. For example, in 1934 Ferguson wrote:

> Our spines were developed for the four-footed position and are not yet adapted to the erect, so mechanical weakness at the lumbosacral area is usual rather than exceptional. We must consider the lumbosacral area not as normal or abnormal but as mechanically sound or mechanically unsound.[9]

Lumbosacral Facets

Congenital alignment of articular surfaces and mechanical dsyfuntions are best demonstrated at the lumbosacral junction. Without doubt, lumbosacral joint asymmetry is associated with a higher incidence of low back pain, and the pain is more difficult to treat than when the two joints are similar in orientation (Fig. 2). The normal lumbosacral joint is in the coronal plane. This orientation allows the joint to

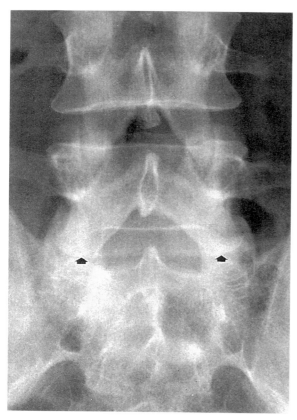

FIGURE 2. The normal lumbosacral facets (closed arrows) should have a coronal orientation. This orientation allows for flexion, extension, and some sidebending but little rotation.

accommodate flexion and extension and some rotation but not much sidebending (Fig. 3).

Radiographs of the lumbosacral spine reveal many variations of the lumbosacral joints, including inclined, rudimentary, irregular, and defective joints.[22,29] If the lumbosacral joints are more sagittal in orientation, stress on both the ligaments and the lamina is greater.[27] As a result, the downward forces of gravity press the lumbosacral joints together in an abnormal and asymmetric fashion and thereby ac-

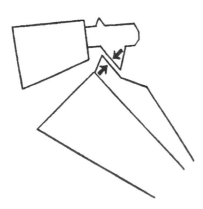

FIGURE 3. "A diagram to indicate the buttress-like (antiluxation) action of the lumbosacral articular processes." This drawing and caption are from Mitchell's 1934 article in the *Journal of Bone and Joint Surgery*.[27]

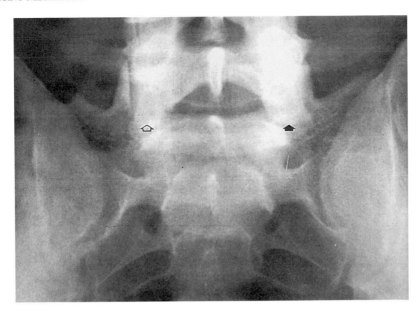

FIGURE 4. The lumbosacral junction commonly has facets of different orientation; one joint has a coronal orientation (closed arrow) and the other is in a more sagittal plane (open arrow). The radiologic assessment of joint orientation can be helpful in the evaluation of low back pain. The patient with asymmetric joints is a likely candidate for mechanical dysfunctions of the lumbosacral junction.

celerate the development of degenerative joint disease. The most common finding is a low back with asymmetric lumbosacral joints, one coronal and one sagittal (Fig. 4). This situation is a functional disaster, and it is easy to imagine how it can lead to mechanical joint dysfunction. For example, if a person has asymmetric lumbosacral facet alignment, and lifts from the side, one of the joints may well malfunction. Assessment of joint orientation cannot be overemphasized and justifies plain film imaging of the lumbar spine. Ferguson concluded that "practically every person with a severe degree of asymmetry of these facets has symptoms referable to the lower part of the back."[9]

Leg Length and Unlevel Sacral Base

The effect of leg length on mechanical dysfunction has been the subject of articles for nearly a hundred years. Controversies have waxed and waned about the importance of leg-length discrepancies and whether it is fair to call them a congenital anomaly since they are so common.[25] Leg length is just a part of the problem; what really matters is what happens to the sacral base. Is the sacral base level? That is the crucial question. The entire rear quarter is frequently smaller, including the ipsilateral sacral ala, ilium, and leg. The actual measurement of leg length is only one component of the total difference. The impact of this anomaly on mechanical dysfunctions of the back seems directly related to the degree of an unlevel sacral base (Fig. 5). The unlevel sacral base creates joint dysfunctions in the pelvis, such as sacral shears and torsion, and long- and short-curve scoliosis in the axial skeleton.

Does an unlevel sacral base treated with foot lifts alter low back pain? The results of such treatment have been unpredictable. Several authors[3,17,24] have pointed

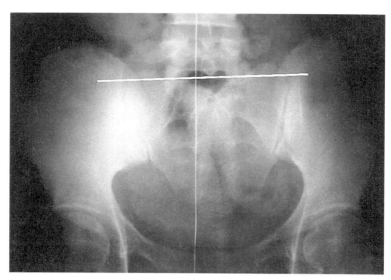

FIGURE 5. The assessment of the level sacral base is an important part of the standing anteroposterior film of the pelvis. The amount of sacral base leveling usually involves more than just the leg-length difference. The size of the ipsilateral sacral ala and the ilium also affects the degree of sacral base leveling. An unlevel sacral base may create numerous mechanical dysfunctions that involve the lumbar spine, lumbosacral junction, sacroiliac joint, and even the hip. The white vertical line is a true vertical wire.

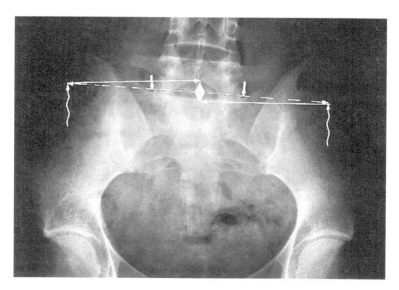

FIGURE 6. Calculation of degree of sacral base unleveling. First find the lateral sacral notches (solid arrows) and draw a line connecting them and extend it over the femoral heads (dashed line). Draw two vertical lines from the apex of the femoral heads to meet the dashed line representing the sacral base inclination (wavy vertical lines). Next draw two horizontal lines (solid lines) across the film that intersect the sacral base line at the femoral heads. The amount of foot lift necessary to correct the sacral base leveling is the distance in millimeters between the two solid lines (diamond).

out that in some patients the treatment of leg-length differences is an effective, simple, and inexpensive way to decrease low back pain. An unlevel sacral base can be corrected mechanically by "foot lifts." Figure 6 illustrates how to calculate the amount of lift necessary to achieve a level sacral base. The first step is to calculate the degree of unlevelness of the sacral base by drawing a line that connects the lateral sacral notches and extending it over the femoral heads. The next step is to draw two vertical lines from the apex of the femoral heads to the line representing the sacral base inclination. The final step is to draw two horizontal lines, each of which intersects the sacral base line at the femoral heads. The amount of foot lift necessary to correct the unleveling is the distance in millimeters between the two horizontal lines.

An unlevel sacral base seems to need some form of corrective curve; however, much of the correction often occurs at the level of the lumbosacral junction and L4. If the sacrum is unlevel to one side, a compensatory sidebending and rotation of L4 or L5 relative to S1 helps to correct the sacral base tilt. Identifying the sidebending and rotation is often not as difficult radiographically as one may imagine (Fig. 7).

Frymoyer[14] and others have noted that such radiographic findings are often present in patients who have no back pain; they do not indicate that the patient's back hurts. However, in patients with back pain, such findings are important. They can aid in defining the amount of lift needed to correct the dysfunction, but whether the lift will work can be determined only by clinical trial and error.

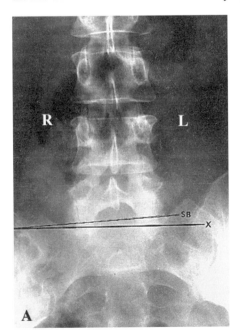
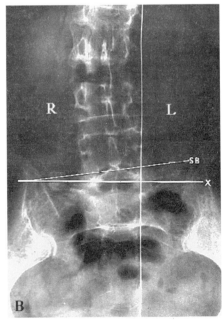

FIGURE 7. *A*, slight abnormal sacral base leveling may create mechanical dysfunctions at the L4 and L5 levels. The line X is horizontal. *B*, line SB is the sacral base axis in the coronal plane. This forces L5 to sidebend to the left and to rotate to the left. Short-curve scoliosis is part of the compensatory changes to the unlevel sacrum. Greater degrees of an unlevel sacral base require a compensatory curve of the entire lumbar spine.

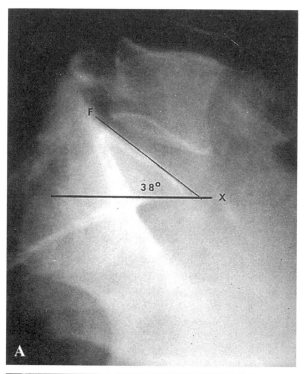

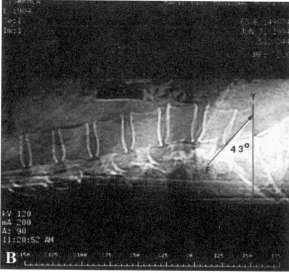

FIGURE 8. Ferguson's angle changes between lying and standing and is not a fixed angle. In fact, it can help to establish the presence of low back pain, as in this case. The angles should increase between horizontal and vertical (see Fig. 9). *A*, in the standing image, line x is horizontal. *B*, in the supine image, line y is vertical. The MR image is a convenient way to get a true supine measurement of Ferguson's angle. The lines labeled F are drawn along the cephalad surface of S1 in both images. In the normal individual this angle increases 4–7° when the patient is standing. In the painful low back the angle decreases as in this case.

Ferguson's Angle

Because the lumbosacral junction is unique in each patient, assessment with the lateral radiograph reveals considerable information about the workings of the lumbar spine. The line developed between the true horizontal and the cephalad surface of the first sacral vertebra is known as Ferguson's angle. This angle is seldom

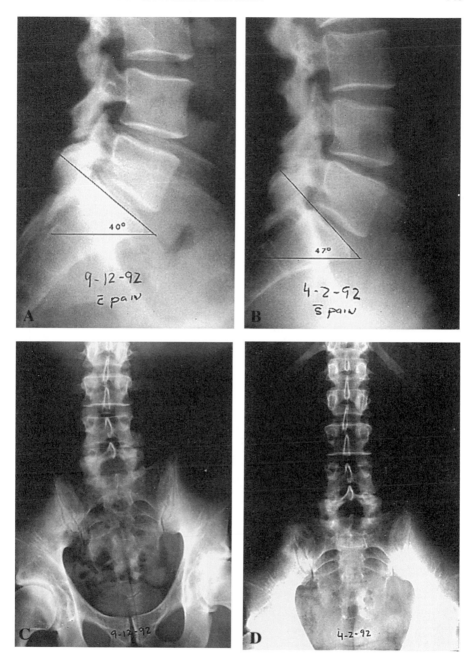

FIGURE 9. The spine changes appearance between the painful and nonpainful states in both the anteroposterior and lateral planes. Notice that on the lateral (*A* and *B*) lumbar spine films, Ferguson's angle is less when the patient was in pain (*A*). In the anteroposterior plane (*C*, with pain, and *D*, without pain) notice the change in the apparent scoliosis.

measured, but it is worth the effort. Ferguson documented that the angle changes between horizontal and vertical radiographic imaging. He also noted that the sacrum moves with gravitational stress and that the movement is different in patients with low back pain. Some paradoxical movement of the sacrum has been confirmed clinically in patients with low back pain by use of the Levator.[23] In normal individuals, Ferguson's angle increases; in patients with low back pain, the sacrum moves into extension, and the angle decreases[12] (Figs. 8 and 9).

The normal horizontal lumbosacral angle is about 42°. If it is greater than 52°, the shear stresses at the lumbosacral junction become significant. Steep angles combined with abnormal lumbosacral joints are functionally unstable. Facet blocks may be diagnostic and helpful in patients with central back pain.

LIGAMENT LAXITY

Ligament laxity, which is believed by many to be one of the primary causes of persistent mechanical dysfunctions, may create numerous radiographic findings in both the cervical and lumbar spine. The demonstration of cervical ligamentous laxity after severe trauma was once the major reason for plain radiographs of the cervical spine; it is now a lost art. Magnetic resonance (MR) and computed tomography (CT) scanners are not as useful for demonstrating ligamentous laxity after an accident as ordinary radiographs with the patient standing in the anteroposterior, lateral neutral, flexion, and extension positions. The plain films demonstrate laxity from the apical ligaments to the lumbosacral spine.

The ligaments that stabilize the occiput, atlas, and axis are particularly vulnerable during whiplash-type injuries. The apical ligaments fix the odontoid to the base of the skull on the edge of the foramen magnum. The transverse ligament stabilizes C1 in relation to C2. Laxity of these ligaments is often demonstrated on plain films.

The open-mouth odontoid-view best demonstrates laxity of the apical ligaments. If the odontoid is not perfectly centered between the lateral masses of the atlas, laxity of the apical ligaments can be inferred (Fig. 10).

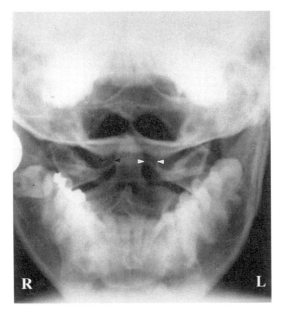

FIGURE 10. Ligament laxities in the spine may occur from the apical ligaments to the sacroiliac joints. This open-mouth odontoid view illustrates laxity of the apical ligaments, which span the space between the apex of the odontoid and the base of the skull at the foreman magnum. The odontoid should be seen equally between the lateral masses of C1 in the normal individual; when they are lax, the odontoid appears asymmetric between the lateral masses of C1. In this film the distance between the white arrows is greater than between the black arrows.

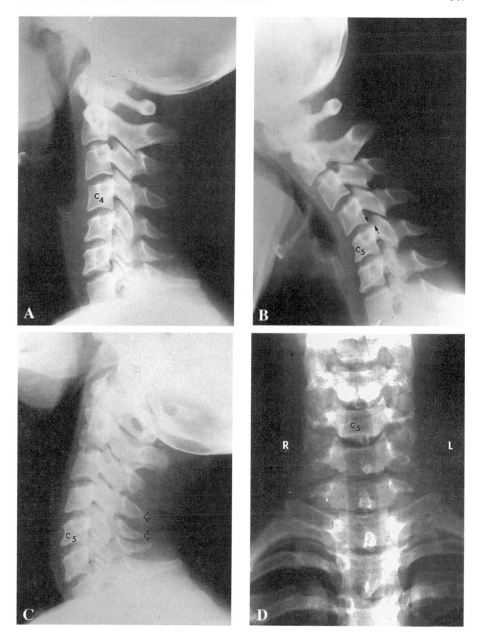

FIGURE 11. Typical whiplash-type injury in a standing cervical spine series. The lateral neutral (*A*) view reveals that C4 is stuck in flexion, creating a reverse lordosis. In flexion, the lateral film demonstrates anterior subluxation of C4 on C5 (*B*). The extension film reveals that the spinous process of C4 does not approach the C5 spinous process, as it should in normal extension (open arrows). C4 and C5 are fixed in flexion and will not move into extension. The anteroposterior view (*D*) demonstrates the presence of mechanical dysfunctions of C4 and C5, which are sidebent to the left. The mechanical dyfunctions of C4 and C5 are described as flexed, sidebent left, and rotated left.

The ligaments and capsules of the zygapophyseal joints are important for stabilization of the neck in flexion and extension. These ligaments are particularly vulnerable during whiplash-type injuries. Vertebral body translation—anterior, posterior, or both—is a reflection of ligamentous laxity. A lateral flexion view of the cervical spine may demonstrate anterior subluxation (Fig. 11).

Lumbar ligamentous laxity allows increased motion of the lumbar vertebrae upon each other. This finding, often noted on lateral films, may be justification for fusion. Figure 12 shows an example of considerable ligamentous laxity at L5–S1. This type of degenerative spondylosis represents the true endpoint of ligamentous laxity of the lumbosacral structures.

ACQUIRED SOMATIC JOINT DYSFUNCTIONS

Radiography of the cervical and lumbar spines may demonstrate persistent mechanical joint dysfunctions. Recent literature reconfirms Jackson's findings of 25 years ago that the trauma of a whiplash-type injury leads to persistent mechanical dysfunctions and subtle but real radiographic findings.[1,7]

The radiographic evaluation of the lumbar spine for somatic joint dysfunctions has remained a challenge since the first osteopaths began to evaluate these structures radiographically in the early 1900s. The difficulty has been the correlation of physical examination of a specific mechanical joint dysfunction with a specific radiographic finding. Such correlations pose a terrific challenge to both hand and eye and frequently are likened to the prestidigitation of magicians. The problem is that the radiologic observers of such changes have little or no ability to evaluate clinically the presence of mechanical joint dysfunctions and vice versa.

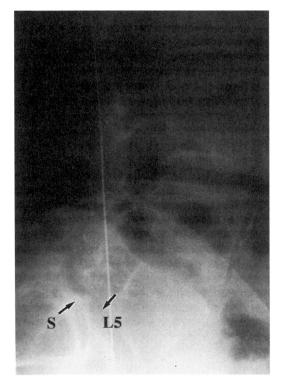

FIGURE 12.   Lateral lumbar spine demonstrating degenerative spondyloses of L5 on S1 (open arrow). This is the ultimate in ligamentous laxity.

TABLE 1. Characteristic Changes of Vertebral Dysfunction

	Position	Motion
C4 on C5 or L4 on L5	Flexed, left-rotated	Extension, right rotation
	Left-sidebent	Right sidebending
	Extended	Flexion
	Right-rotated	Left rotation
	Left-sidebent	Right sidebending

Common cervical radiographic features of whiplash-type injuries are loss of lordosis and a persistently sidebent vertebra. L3, L4, and L5 are frequently involved in radiographic demonstrations of mechanical dysfunctions. A review of the basic findings of mechanical dysfunctions in the cervical and lumbar spine is in order.

The radiographic description should follow the palpatory findings, as defined by Greenman.[17] In current convention vertebral dysfunction is described either by the position of the restricted segment or by the motion that is lost in the restricted segment. Therefore, a segment that is backward-bent (extended), right-rotated, and right-sidebent has lost the motion of forward bending (flexion), left sidebending, and left rotation. Rotation is defined as the direction in which the anterior surface of the vertebral body points. Table 1 summarizes the changes.

Occiput

The mechanical dysfunctions of C1 created by the typical whiplash-type injury are frequent causes of headaches. The usual four-view examination of the normal cervical spine—anteroposterior, neutral lateral, flexion, and extension—should demonstrate movement of C1. In flexion, the distance between the occiput and the posterior aspects of C1 should increase. In extension, the occiput, C1, and the spinous process of C2 should be nearly touching. Figure 10 contrasts normal movement of C1 and C2 with abnormal movement of C4 and C5.

A C1 vertebra fixed in extension or unable to move into flexion is demonstrated in Figure 13. Note that between the flexion and extension views the relationships between the C1 and C2 vertebral bodies and their spinous processes does not change. In this case the relative lack of movement is between the vertebral bodies, but just as frequently the relationship of C1 with the occiput does not change. The space between the occiput and the spinous processes of C1, C2, and C3 should increase during flexion and nearly disappear during extension. However, in this example there is no relative movement of the two vertebral bodies.

Middle and Lower Cervical Spine

Mechanical dysfunctions of the middle and lower cervical vertebrae are perhaps even more common than those of the lumbar spine, although statistical evidence is lacking. The isolated vertebra fixed in flexion or extension with some persistent sidebending is a common finding on many standing cervical spine films of patients with whiplash-type injuries. The frequently noted "straight" cervical spine with loss of lordosis represents the classic mechanical dysfunction. In neutral (Fig. 11A) C4 shows loss of normal lordosis. In fact, the upper four vertebrae appear to be in reverse lordosis. A closer look at Figure 11A reveals that the C4 vertebra is fixed in flexion; that is, it will not go into extension and the neck remains straight. In cervical flexion (Fig. 11B) the C4 vertebra normally moves forward and in fact subluxes slightly on C5 because of ligamentous laxity. Note that in normal flexion the spinous processes appear to fan out equally.

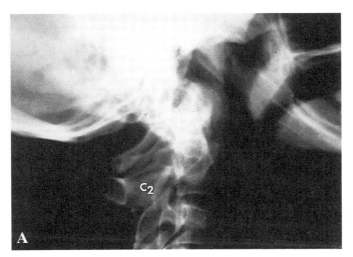

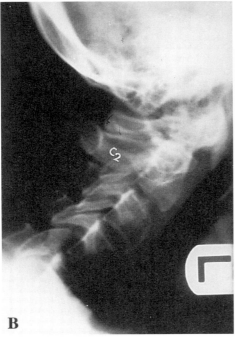

FIGURE 13. A mechanical joint dysfunction of the atlas on the axis. Notice that there is no relative movement between the two vertebrae between maximal extension (*A*) and flexion (*B*). In flexion, C1 should open up relative to C2. In this example, compare the movement of C1 with the movement of C1 in Figure 10. Mechanical joint dysfunctions involving the occiput (C1, C2, and C3) are common clinically and often show radiographic changes in a functional cervical spine series.

In the extension film (Fig. 11C), the C4 vertebra that is fixed in flexion and does not go into extension is identified by the gap between the spinous process of C4 and C5.

The anteroposterior film of the cervical spine (Fig. 11D) demonstrates short curve scoliosis and asymmetry in the joint spaces of Luschka at C4 and C5. This finding is also evidence of mechanical dysfunctions of the cervical vertebrae. Another example of this type of mechanical dysfunction is demonstrated in Figure 14, a neutral anteroposterior film of the cervical spine. This film reveals some sidebending at C4 and C5. Note the asymmetry in the joints of Luschka between the

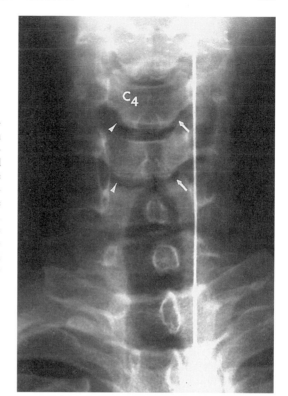

FIGURE 14. Short-curve scoliosis in the anteroposterior projection is a sign of mechanical dysfunctions. In this cervical spine, C4 and C5 are sidebent to the left. Notice that the left joints of Luschka (arrows) are closer together on the joints on the right (arrowheads). The vertebrae are also rotated to the left. In the cervical spine, sidebending and rotation are coupled movements and almost always go together.

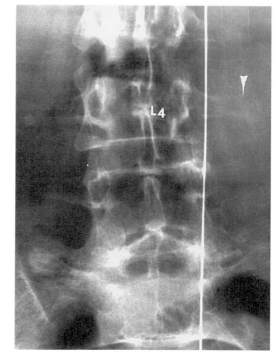

FIGURE 15. Mechanical joint dysfunction of the fourth lumbar vertebra (L4). The vertebra is sidebent to the left and rotated to the right. The rotation can be seen in the appearance of the transverse processes. In this case the left transverse process has rotated into the plane of the film (arrowhead). This mechanical dysfunction is manipulable. One can frequently find tracks of mechanical joint dysfunctions on all types of lumbar images. Rotation of the vertebra is defined as the direction in which the anterior aspect of the vertebral body moves.

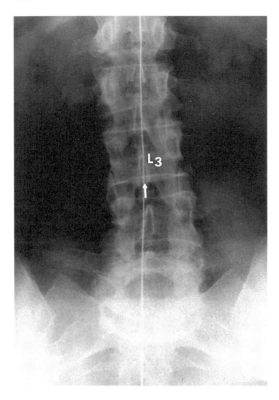

FIGURE 16. The L3 vertebra is sidebent to the right and rotated to the left, and the L3 spinous process (arrow) appears to be on the right side of the vertebral body. Mechanical joint dysfunctions of L2 and L3 are common and frequently visualized on radiography of the lumbosacral spine. Clinically they are often involved in mechanical dysfunctions. Their attachments to the psoas muscle cause them to be flexed and sidebent to the side of the psoas spasm. In contrast to the cervical spine, their motions may not be coupled so that they may rotate to one side and sidebend to the other, i.e., rotate to the left and sidebend to the right.

right and left sides. Note also that C4 is rotated to the left and that the shadow of the spinous process appears to be more on the right side of the vertebra than on the left. In the cervical spine, the coupled motions of sidebending and rotation are nearly always seen together.

Lumbar Vertebrae

Mechanical dysfunctions of the pelvis and lumbar spine leave numerous radiographic findings. The persistently sidebent and rotated L4 or L5 vertebra is often seen on both plain film and computer-aided images. Sidebending in the lumbar spine is easy to see on radiography, because the transverse processes are closer together on one side than on the other (Fig. 15). Sidebending often comes with rotation, in either an ipsilateral or contralateral direction, because in spinal joints the two movements are coupled (Fig. 16).

To complete the diagnosis of mechanical joint dysfunction, flexion, extension, and sidebending images are helpful. Lateral flexion and extension views may demonstrate whether the vertebra moves normally in the sagittal plane. The movements are like those in the cervical spine but much more subtle. Neutral lateral, flexion, and extension images demonstrate an extended L3 (Fig. 17). The lateral lumbar spine appears grossly normal with the exception of apparent hyperlordosis (Fig. 17A). The spine looks normal in extension because the spinous processes close together normally (Fig. 17B). Note the resistance of the L3 vertebra to flexion, which gives the appearance of a flat back during the attempt at flexion (Fig. 17C). The limited flexion of L3 is also due in part to natural lordosis. In clinical practice this type

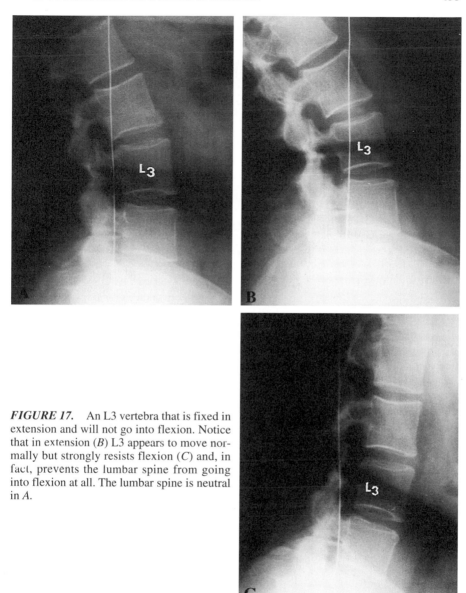

FIGURE 17.   An L3 vertebra that is fixed in extension and will not go into flexion. Notice that in extension (B) L3 appears to move normally but strongly resists flexion (C) and, in fact, prevents the lumbar spine from going into flexion at all. The lumbar spine is neutral in A.

of radiographic demonstration adds little to the treatment protocol and almost nothing to the palpatory findings.

Sacroiliac Joints

Changes in the sacroiliac joints, although commonly seen on both plain and MR/CT images, are not usually viewed as reflecting mechanical dysfunction. Over the years, however numerous authors have commented that such changes may be degenerative.[5] Osteophytes, subarticular sclerosis (osteitis condenses), and joint

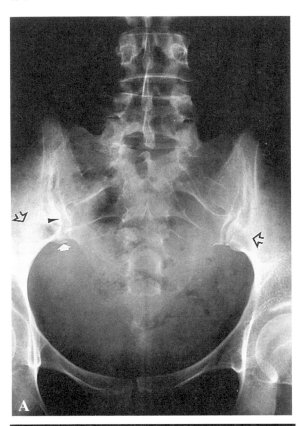

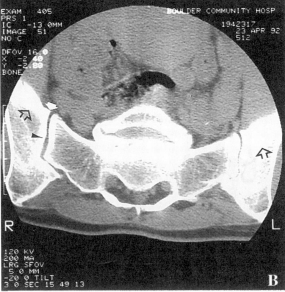

FIGURE 18. Degenerative joint disease of the sacroiliac joint is a common radiographic finding on both plain film and MR/CT imaging. An anteroposterior pelvic plain film (*A*) and CT scan (*B*) demonstrate joint space widening on the right (arrowheads), inferior osteophytes (closed white arrows), and osteitis condenses illi (closed black arrows). These radiographic changes are signs of mechanical dysfunctions of the joint and deserve to be commented on routinely.

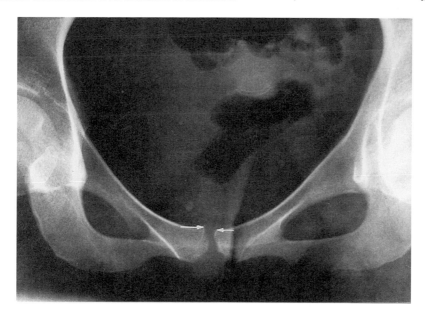

FIGURE 19.   Pubic dysfunctions are often demonstrated on the standing pelvic radiograph. The two pubes should be equal in height. When the pubic rami are not aligned symmetrically (arrows), one can deduce the presence of mechanical dysfunction. Which half of the pelvis is abnormal is a clinical diagnosis.

space narrowing indicate abnormal joint mechanics (Fig. 18). The developing consensus is that such findings on all forms of imaging represent mechanical joint dysfunctions and ligamentous laxity[6] and provide excellent documentation when correlated with clinical findings.[18]

Symphysis Pubis

Mechanical dysfunction of the symphysis pubis is a common clinical diagnosis. The alignment of the pubic bones is critical in diagnosis and treatment of mechanical dysfunction of the pelvis. Ilial upslip, downslip, and rotation are easily identified clinically and create characteristic radiographic changes. The demonstration of symphysis pubis dysfunctions on plain x-ray films is also common (Fig. 19). Evaluation of the symphysis pubis on anteroposterior pelvic image aids in the documentation of displacement and is of considerable help to the treating clinician. It is critical to obtain such images with the patient standing.

The three bones and joints of the pelvis work in unison, and dysfunction of one joint leads to instability in the entire structure, just as the uncoupling of one angle destabilizes a triangle. Treatment of pelvic dysfunction, therefore, begins with treatment of the symphysis pubis.

The radiographic manifestation of mechanical dysfunction of the symphysis pubis is simply malalignment of the two pubic bones. This finding is sometimes considered to be positional but most often results from a true mechanical dysfunction of the pelvis. Pubic displacements, combined with degenerative disease of the sacroiliac joints, are further evidence of sacroiliac mechanical dysfunction.

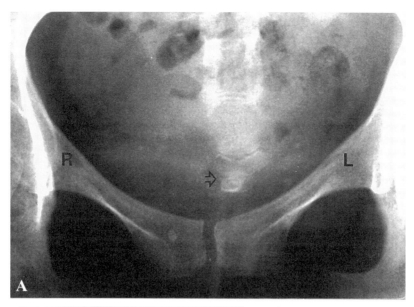

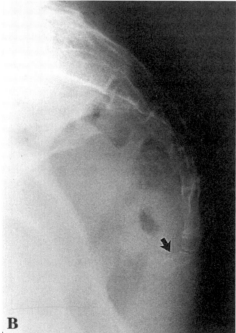

FIGURE 20. The coccyx, an important bone in the low back, is easily seen on the anteroposterior films of the pelvis (*A*), but on the lateral pelvic images it may be hard to identify (*B*). It is usually forced into abnormal flexion (closed arrow). Mechanical dysfunctions of the coccyx can cause diverse clinical problems, including headaches, low back pain, and even incontinence.

Coccyx

The coccyx is a small bone often ignored on imaging, but it is a vital link between the bony pelvis and soft tissues of the pelvic floor.[2] The human coccyx is the tail that is capable of wagging the body. The coccyx has direct attachments to the sacrotuberous ligaments and the dural sac through the filum terminale. Mechanical dysfunctions of this small bone may affect the axial skeleton directly by way of its connection to the dura as well as create visceral dysfunctions by straining all of the muscles and ligamentous structures of the pelvic floor. Somatic joint dysfunctions include difficult-to-treat low back pain, headaches, and even incontinence in women.

The coccyx is usually forced into excessive flexion. It is a vulnerable structure in many thin people, particularly those without gluteal muscle mass. Radiographic demonstrations of mechanical displacements of the coccyx are helpful because such displacements are often hard to identify clinically and may be overlooked (Fig. 20).

COMPUTERIZED IMAGING AND MECHANICAL DYSFUNCTIONS

Sacral Torsion (Asymlocation)

A number of somatic dysfunctions can be identified on MRI/CT scanning. The most common is sacral torsion, which can be thought of as a sacrum with simultaneous mechanical dysfunctions in sidebending, flexion, or extension. This disorder is possible because of the unique nature of the sacroiliac joints. The basic model of spinal mechanics suggests that sidebending and rotation are integral parts of spinal and sacral motion. The normal sacrum lies horizontal in a gantry and should be nearly parallel with the floor. If a sidebent lesion is present anywhere in the spine, the most likely place for torsion to be exhibited is at the level of the involved vertebra. However, torsion occasionally manifests as rotation at either end of the spine (sacrum or atlas).[16] This sacral twisting is often evident on MRI/ CT scans. In normal patients without mechanical joint dysfunctions the spine is straight. In patients with one or more vertebral somatic joint dysfunctions that are sidebent and rotated, the spine is curved. This curve or kink in the spine creates a twisting that travels to both ends. The twisting of the sacrum is not created by malposition of the patient but by mechanical dysfunction (Fig. 21). If sacral torsion is mechanically corrected by forcing the sacrum into a horizontal plane, the patient quickly becomes uncomfortable, because the spine is forced to sidebend. The patient eventually finds a more comfortable position by rotating the spine to undo the sidebending.

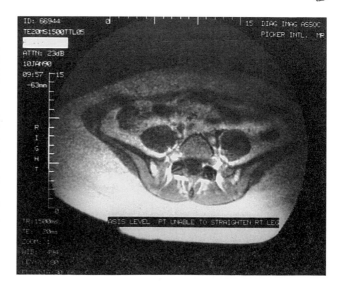

FIGURE 21. Sacral torsion (asymlocation) or twisting is a frequent finding on MR/CT images of the low back. Sacral torsion may be a consequence of proximal mechanical dysfunctions of the spine or an isolated lesion. This MRI demonstrates left rotation of the sacrum. Note that the anterior iliac spines are level, but the sacrum is rotated to the left.

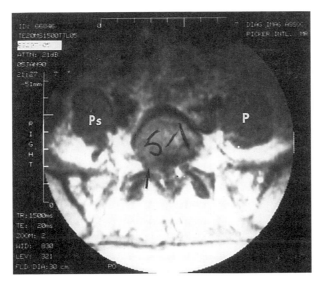

FIGURE 22. Lumbar MR/CT scans often reveal asymmetric psoas muscles (P). This asymmetry may be the result of unilateral psoas muscle spasm (right; Ps). The spasm is capable of creating lumbar spinal compression and sidebending, both of which may cause the disk to bulge (arrow). Psoas muscle spasm can create numerous mechanical dysfunctions and pain in the lumbosacral spine; it should be clinically evaluated in patients with low back pain.

Sacral torsion is quite common in patients with back pain, and close examination of the MRI/CT scan often reveals sacral torsion to one degree or another. At this point the normal range of sacral torsion on MRI/CT is unknown, but the gross changes noted on many scans are clearly abnormal. Radiographic evidence of sacral torsion may be helpful in the diagnosis of lumbosacral mechanical dysfunctions.

Disk Bulging

"Disk bulging" is a somewhat surprising term, particularly when the MRI/CT scan demonstrates that the vertebra either above or below the involved disk is both sidebent and rotated to the side of the bulge. The result is a much narrower disk space on the affected side. This cause for a "bulging disk" is seldom, if ever, acknowledged. The importance of disk bulging noted on MRI/CT scan remains controversial,[21] and most instances may well result from localized somatic joint dysfunction, particularly when the bulging is unilateral. The distance between the radiographer and the clinician is clear in the "bulging disk" scenario.

Another common cause for a bulging disk is muscle spasm.[26] Because of its size, position, and strength, the psoas muscle is capable of compressing all of the lumbar intervertebral disks (Fig. 22). Asymmetry between the psoas muscles, as seen on computerized imaging, is often ignored because it is hard to quantify. Clinically spasm of the psoas muscle may create some degree of scoliosis, and the muscle mass pulls away from the spine on the side of the spasm. The clinical findings of psoas spasm should be correlated with radiographic findings. Changes in the cross sectional area and even muscle density, which are evident on the images, may be of considerable clinical importance. The many clinical problems created by the psoas muscle merit a complete chapter.

Ligament Laxity

Although MRI has offered new opportunities to illustrate ligament integrity, its use to evaluate lumbosacral ligamentous laxity is yet to come. Abnormal MRI findings in major structures such as the Achilles tendon, patellar tendon, and anterior

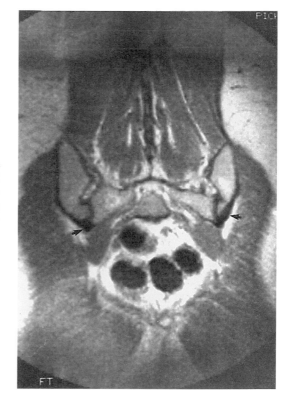

FIGURE 23. MRI coronal image of the pelvis demonstrates normal lower sacroiliac ligaments (arrows). The usefulness of imaging the pelvic ligaments with MRI remains to be demonstrated.

cruciate ligament are now recognized as diagnostic of ligamentous injury. The same findings have not been so clearly demonstrated in the iliolumbar and upper and lower sacroiliac ligaments, but careful observation and study may demonstrate similar changes (Fig. 23).

THE RADIOLOGIC CLINICIAN

Fifty years ago many radiologists clearly understood the clinical importance of their images because they worked with internists and surgeons in back pain clinics, evaluating and treating patients. Early radiologists developed palpatory skills that allowed them to understand altered function and imaging skills that improved the diagnosis. More recently, the usefulness of the radiographic image has been questioned. It has been stated and restated that radiographic abnormalities are present in patients who have no back pain and that such findings do not indicate that the patient's back hurts. The patients in these often quoted studies were not evaluated for mechanical dysfunctions or ligament pain; at most the physical examination was limited to a few neurologic and range-of-motion tests.

The evaluation of low back pain by radiologists can be of considerable aid to the clinician and support therapeutic efforts. Lesions often may be present but not painful. On the other hand, lesions may be painful and respond to treatment without radiographic change. The reason for finding such lesions radiographically is to make the clinician aware of anatomic conditions and mechanical problems that need clinical correlation. Let the radiologic clinician return to the evaluation of low back pain in the clinic and in the x-ray room.

SUMMARY

Acquired mechanical somatic joint dysfunctions, such as the persistently sidebent and rotated cervical or lumbar vertebra, are commonly seen on all types of images of the spine. They are also common causes of neck and back pain. Identification by imaging is important, because treatment by manipulation may depend on radiologic documentation.

The orientation of the lumbosacral facets is best evaluated with plain films. Congenital anomalies may create important clinical problems. The normal coronal facets are associated with fewer clinical problems than facets of other orientation. An unlevel sacral base, as seen on the anteroposterior pelvic film, may explain the resistance of a mechanical joint dysfunction to manipulation. The correction of an unlevel sacral base can be determined by measurements taken from the radiographs. Ferguson's angle, often viewed as a static measure, is in fact dynamic and changes paradoxically in the painful low back. Sacroiliac joints showing changes of degenerative disease may reflect longstanding mechanical dysfunction.

The identification of a malaligned symphysis pubis and degenerative sacroiliac disease can be of considerable service to the clinician struggling with an "unstable back." A coccyx in an excessively flexed position can help to explain pelvic and back pain that seems to have no explanation.

Computerized imaging can identify both congenital and acquired dysfunctions, such as sacral torsion and sacral sidebent lesions. The common "disk bulge" is frequently associated with mechanical joint dysfunctions of the sacrum and lumbar spine. The identification of disk bulging by radiograph should carry with it observations about adjacent mechanical joint dysfunctions.

It may be unfair at this point to ask radiologists to evaluate the images of patients with the above findings. Their ability to do so may be limited by their understanding of spinal mechanics. The radiographic literature of the past 50 years contains only a handful of articles relevant to the relationships between images and mechanical dysfunctions—and some of these are not supportive. Contemporary spinal diagnostic and therapeutic literature emphasizes imaging of the disks. Radiologists who understand the congenital and mechanical dysfunctions of the cervical and lumbosacral spine and their importance to the clinician can help to bridge the gap.

REFERENCES

 1. Barnsley L: The prevalence of chronic cervical zygapophyseal joint pain after whiplash. Spine 20:20–26, 1995.
 2. Barral JP: Visceral Manipulation. Seattle, Eastland Press, 1988.
 3. Denslow JS: Mechanical stresses in the human lumbar spine and pelvis (1962). In Postural Balance and Imbalance. Indianapolis, American Academy of Osteopathy, 1983.
 4. Denslow JS: Methods in taking and interpreting weightbearing x-ray films. J Am Osteopath Assoc 54:663–670, 1955.
 5. Dilhman W: Diagnostic Radiology of the Sacroiliac Joints. New York, Georg Thieme, 1980.
 6. Dreyfuss P: The sacroiliac joint: A review. Isis 2:22–58, 1994.
 7. Dvorak J: Functional radiographic diagnosis of the cervical spine: Flexion/extension. Spine 13:748–755, 1988.
 8. Farfan HF: The relationship of facet orientation to intervertebral disc failure. Can J Surg 10:179–185, 1967.
 9. Ferguson AB: The clinical and roentgenographic interpretation of lumbosacral anomalies. Radiology 22:548–588, 1934.
10. [Reference deleted].
11. Fortin JD: Sacroiliac joint dysfunction—a new perspective. J Back Musculoskel Rehabil 3:31–43, 1993.

12. Frisch H: Systematic Musculoskeletal Examination. New York, Springer-Verlag, 1994.
13. Fryette HH: Some reasons why SI lesions recur. J Am Osteopath Assoc 36:119–122, 1936.
14. Frymoyer JW: Spine radiographs in patients with low back pain. J Bone Joint Surg 66A:1048–1055, 1984.
15. [Reference deleted].
16. Gracovetsky S: The Spinal Engine. New York, Springer-Verlag, 1988.
17. Greenman PE: Principles of Manual Medicine. Baltimore, Williams & Wilkins, 1989.
18. Greenman PE: Sacroiliac dysfunction in the failed low back pain syndrome. In Proceedings for the First Interdisciplinary World Congress on Low Back Pain and Its Relation to the Sacroiliac Joint. San Diego, 1992, pp 329–352.
19. Hagg O: Facet joint asymmetry and protrusion of the intervertebral disc. Spine 15:356–359, 1990.
20. Jackson R: The Cervical Syndrome. Springfield, IL, Charles C. Thomas, 1977.
21. Jensen MC: Magnetic resonance imaging of the lumbar spine in people without back pain. N Engl J Med 331:69–73, 1994.
22. Jonsson B: Anomalous lumbosacral articulations and low-back pain—Evaluation and treatment. Spine 14:831–834, 1989.
23. Jungmann M: Backaches, Postural Decline, Aging and Gravity-Strain. New York, Institute for Gravitational Strain Pathology, 1988.
24. Kappler RE: Postural balance and motion patterns. In Postural Balance and Imbalance. Indianapolis, American Academy of Osteopathy, 1983.
25. Kerr HE: Observations on anatomical short leg in a series of patients presenting themselves for treatment of low-back pain. J Am Osteopathic Assoc 42:437–440, 1913.
26. Kuchera W: Osteopathic Principles in Practice. Kirksville, MO, KCOM Press, 1991.
27. Mitchell GAG: The lumbosacral junction. J Bone Joint Surg 16:233–254, 1934.
28. Twomey L: Spine update: Exercise and spinal manipulation in the treatment of low back pain. Spine 20:615–619, 1995.
29. Van Schaik JPJ: The orientation of laminae and facet joints in the lower lumbar spine. Spine 10:59–63, 1985.

MICHAEL L. KUCHERA, DO, FAAO

GRAVITATIONAL STRESS, MUSCULOLIGAMENTOUS STRAIN, AND POSTURAL ALIGNMENT

From the Department of
  Osteopathic Manipulative
  Medicine
Kirksville College of Osteopathic
  Medicine
Kirksville, Missouri

Reprint requests to:
Michael L. Kuchera, DO, FAAO
Professor and Chairman
Department of Osteopathic
  Manipulative Medicine
Kirksville College of Osteopathic
  Medicine
800 West Jefferson
Kirksville, MO 63501

If we regard posture as the result of the dynamic interaction of two groups of forces—the environmental force of gravity on one hand, and the strength of the individual on the other—then posture is but the formal expression of the balance of power existing at any time between these two groups of forces. Thus, any deterioration of posture indicates that the individual is losing ground in his contest with the environmental force of gravity.—Martin Jungmann, MD[21]

Gravitational force is a constant and greatly underestimated stressor of the somatic system. This chapter discusses its effect on muscle, ligaments, and other fasciae and the relationship of each to posture and skeletal alignment.

The most obvious effect of gravitational stress can be evaluated by careful observation of posture, which is both static and dynamic. The static alignment of body mass with respect to gravity is constantly adjusted by dynamic neuromuscular coordination as the individual changes position. Over time, individual static postural alignment conforms to inherent connective tissue structure as well as the cumulative functional demands of both static and dynamic postural conditions. Musculoligamentous function is also significantly influenced by, as well as responsible for, static and dynamic postural alignment. Analysis of postural alignment of regions of the body in the upright weightbearing position and orthopedic examination of the selective tensions of the soft tissues provide clinical clues to the inherent ability of the neuromusculoskeletal system to balance and maintain biomechanical alignment.

SPINE: State of the Art Reviews—Vol. 9, No. 2, May 1995
  Philadelphia, Hanley & Belfus, Inc.

463

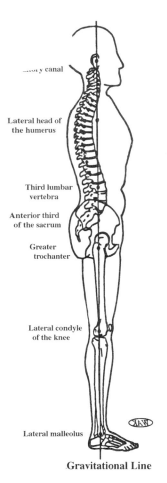

Labels on figure:
...ory canal
Lateral head of the humerus
Third lumbar vertebra
Anterior third of the sacrum
Greater trochanter
Lateral condyle of the knee
Lateral malleolus
Gravitational Line

FIGURE 1. Ideal postural alignment of the body with respect to the gravitational line.

The "ideal" postural alignment (Fig. 1), in which gravitational force is transferred along structures adapted for weightbearing, requires a minimum of energy expenditure by postural muscles and minimal strain on postural ligaments. Maintenance of static and dynamic elements of posture places no additional biomechanical stress on the somatic system.

With less than ideal postural alignment, gravitational force on individual structures is biomechanically amplified[22] and creates additional shearing stress (Fig. 2). Musculoligamentous structures associated with maintenance of posture are thus subjected to increased strain. When the viscoelastic deformative properties of muscle, restraining ligaments, and other connective tissues are unable to resist the stress, neuromuscular reflex activity is initiated automatically and subconsciously to maintain postural equilibrium. Continuous gravitational stress results in various combinations of predictable pathophysiologic change, which begins in the connective tissues. It is accentuated and perpetuated by inadequate host compensatory mechanisms.

Postural muscles are adapted structurally to function in the presence of prolonged gravitational stress. They are generally more resistant to fatigue. When their

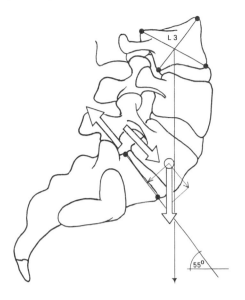

FIGURE 2. Shearing stress increases with anterior weightbearing mechanics (L3 weightbearing line falls anterior to the sacral base), hyperlordosis, and larger lumbosacral or sacral angles. Gravitational stress is transferred to the posterior elements (pars interarticularis), erector spinae muscles, and ligamentous tissues.

capacity to resist stress is overwhelmed, they become irritable, tight, and shortened.[19] Both structural (anatomic) and functional (physiologic and biochemical) changes occur in myofascial structures. They undergo sustained changes in length, and studies[10] suggest that deleterious change is most pronounced in shortened as opposed to lengthened muscles. New collagen, with a half-life of 10–12 months, realigns the connective tissues in response to vectors of stress, thus perpetuating the resultant posture and maintaining biomechanical amplification of gravitational stress. Abnormal stresses, chronically applied to connective tissues, modify their structure and function until they are no longer capable of compensating for the effects of gravitational strain. In an extension of Wolff's law that calcium is laid down along lines of stress, bony exostoses and ligamentous calcification provide radiographic evidence of the stress placed on soft tissue structures and the fibroosseous junction.

When host mechanisms are overwhelmed, signs of gravitational stress appear, including postural decompensation, chronic or recurrent strains and sprains, pseudoparesis, recurrent somatic dysfunction, recurrent myofascial trigger points, and ligamentous laxity. The patient's symptoms include low back pain, pain referred to extremities, headache, fatigue, weakness, dysfunctional symptoms from various viscera, and other sequelae of neural, vascular, and lymphatic dysfunction resulting from somatic stress. The key to efficient diagnosis is to recognize such signs and symptoms as pathophysiologic elements of a common musculoligamentous strain pattern caused by gravitational stress. The treatment plan and prognosis are determined by the physician, who carefully determines the relative degrees of functional disturbance and structural change.

Treatment of patients with musculoligamentous and other somatic dysfunction may incorporate a wide range of therapeutic methods, but for patients in whom gravitational stress is recognized to play a role, postural alignment is vital. Structural and functional goals must be met to achieve appropriate rehabilitation of skeletal, arthrodial, and myofascial elements. Numerous elegant treatment techniques, including manipulation, have proved to be clinically effective. In each technique, afferent in-

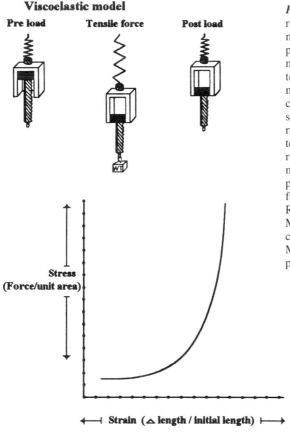

Plastic (viscous model)

Pre load   Tensile force   Post load

Viscoelastic model

Pre load   Tensile force   Post load

Stress
(Force/unit area)

←—| Strain (△ length / initial length) |—→

FIGURE 3. Top row, schematic representation of the viscoelastic model or elongation: plastic component in which deformation remains after the application of tensile force. Middle row, schematic representation of the viscoelastic model of elongation: some elongation is lost and some retained after the application of tensile force. Bottom, graphic representation of viscoelastic deformation: force applied (stress) is plotted against percentage of deformation (strain). (From Cantu RI, Grodin AJ: Myofascial Manipulation: Theory and Clinical Application. Gaithersburg, MD, Aspen Publishers, 1992; with permission.)

formation conveyed to the central nervous system from peripheral receptors in tendons, ligaments, muscle, and other somatic tissue results in a modification of the central response. Muscle reeducation and treatment schemes designed to promote coordinated sequencing of muscle firing are also important. The elements of a complete treatment protocol are developed later in this chapter.

POSTURAL DECOMPENSATION

Gravitational forces are constant, whereas inherent factors vary from individual to individual. Patients with connective tissues disorders such as Ehlers-Danlos syndrome or Ollier's disease have a congenital susceptibility to postural decompensation. Acquired susceptibility is found in patients with ligamentous laxity arising from direct macrotrauma or in patients with biomechanically induced microtrauma. Gravitational stress in susceptible hosts first produces postural compensation. Continued stress typically results in inadequate host resistance and simultaneous decompensation in all three cardinal planes.[32] Postural compensation and decompensation are discussed in reference to the primary plane in which change is maximal. The terms *hyperlordosis* and thoracic *kyphosis* refer to postural disorders in the sagittal plane. *Scoliosis*, postural decompensation in the coronal plane, is often observed in patients with sacral base unleveling. Significant decompensation in the horizontal plane with less coronal plane involvement is more likely to be called *rotoscoliosis*. Certain predictable changes can be seen in the function of musculoligamentous structures as a consequence of gravitational stress-induced pathophysiology, regardless of the plane involved or the posture adopted by the patient.

Numerous authors[1,4,8,17,21,23] have extensively researched posture and the adaptive response of somatic structures to gravitational strain. Muscular dysfunction is especially precipitated and perpetuated in the postural muscles and certain of their antagonists.[19,40,41] The resulting afferent proprioceptive imbalance affects neuromuscular reflex mechanisms associated with maintenance of posture. In general, gravitational stress and the resultant postural effects are more likely to be related to anatomic, histologic, physiologic, and dysfunctional changes at *transitional (junctional) areas* of the spine, which are also predisposed to injury and somatic dysfunction. Thus, spinal somatic dysfunction commonly occurs at craniocervical, cervicothoracic, thoracolumbar, lumbopelvic, and sacroiliac junctions.[6,14,43] The histologic junctional zones created by connective tissue attachments of ligaments, tendons, and joint capsules are also vulnerable to the biomechanical stress of postural decompensation,[2,13] especially for the fibroosseous junction of restraining ligaments.

Connective tissue reaction to stress (Fig. 3) is nonlinear and viscoelastic.[2] The *elastic component* represents a temporary change in connective tissue length in response to stress and is especially important in dynamic postural mechanics. The *viscous component* is responsible for more permanent deformation of connective tissue that occurs in static postural change. Somatic afferent stimulation from receptors in the connective tissue is capable of initiating predictable patterns of referred pain. Ligaments typically create a deep, dull pain in a sclerotomal distribution. Practitioners dealing with the fascial ligamentous system should be familiar with sclerotomal charts (Fig. 4) and ligamentous pain patterns (Fig. 5). Both are essential in understanding gravitational stress-induced pain. Such expertise provides one of the cornerstones of orthopedic medicine. A more detailed description of the ligamentous reaction to stress, including pain pattern distribution and treatment protocols, is found in the definitive text by Hackett.[13]

Both palpatory and radiologic changes are helpful in the diagnosis of ligamentous strain. Chronically stressed ligaments typically undergo progressive change involving the viscous component. The change begins with edema in the region of the fibroosseous junction and tenderness to palpation. Ligamentous laxity eventually occurs. Deposition of calcium frequently follows in a homeostatic attempt to create stability. The deposition of calcium salts along lines of stress produces exostoses at origin and/or insertion of postural muscles and ligaments. Often, calcification of the entire ligament takes place (Fig. 6).

The term *somatic dysfunction* was originally coined by osteopaths to describe the *asymmetry, restricted motion,* and *tissue texture changes* palpable in certain

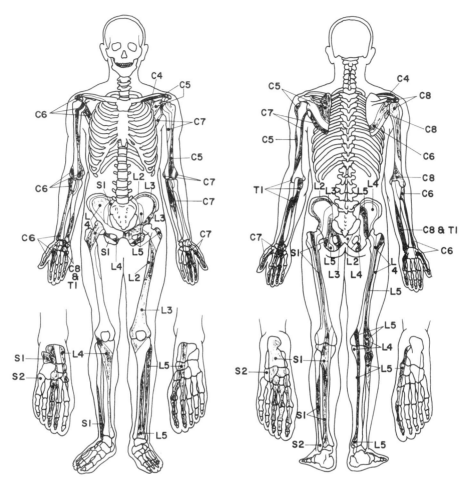

FIGURE 4. Innervation of the skeleton by spinal segments. Sclerotomal pain arising from bone, joint, or ligament is described as deep, dull, "toothache like" pain.

pathophysiologic states. The term has been adopted by orthopedic physicians and is now recognized in the International Classification of Disease as a codable diagnosis by region of the body (739.0–739.9). Somatic dysfunction is specifically defined as "impaired or altered function of somatic tissues—skeletal, arthrodial, and/or myofascial—and its related neural, vascular and lymphatic elements."[7] Early in the process of biomechanical strain, somatic dysfunction often exists alone and is reversible. As structural change is introduced, somatic dysfunction becomes more common, but its treatment restores only a portion of the region's function.

Myofascial dysfunction, including myofascial trigger points, is a specific form of somatic dysfunction with subjective pain and recordable weakness and autonomic and vascular-lymphatic characteristics.[31] Certain muscles react predictably to gravitational stress—not homogeneously, but characteristically for each muscle. Such observations have been described independently by Jungmann,[17,21] Janda,[19] Kuchera,[28] and Travell and Simons.[40,41] In general, postural muscle dysfunction is manifested

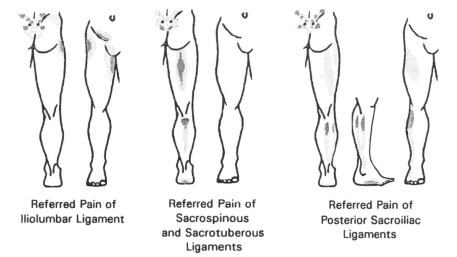

**Referred Pain of
Iliolumbar Ligament**

**Referred Pain of
Sacrospinous
and Sacrotuberous
Ligaments**

**Referred Pain of
Posterior Sacroiliac
Ligaments**

FIGURE 5. Common ligamentous pain patterns arising from gravitational stress and postural malalignment. (Adapted from Hackett GS: Ligament and Tendon Relaxation Treated by Prolotherapy. 3rd ed. Springfield, IL, Charles C. Thomas, 1958.)

by spasm, hypertonicity, and development of myofascial trigger points. Other muscles, especially those antagonistic to the spastic muscles, predictably demonstrate inhibitory characteristics described as pseudoparesis (functional, nonorganic weakness) or myofascial trigger points with weakness.[19,23]

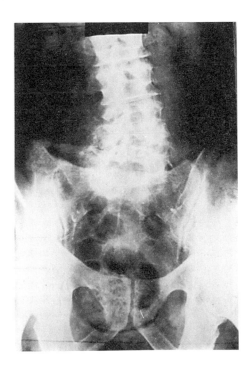

FIGURE 6. Calcification of iliolumbar ligament secondary to postural stress.[21] (From the Institute for Gravitational Strain Pathophysiology, Inc., Rangeley, Maine; with permission.)

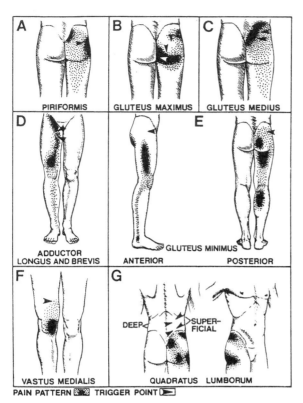

FIGURE 7. Referred pain as documented by Travell and Simons from selected muscles subject to gravity-induced myofascial trigger points. (From Simons DG, Travell JG: Myofascial pain syndromes. In Wall PD, Melzack R (eds): Textbook of Pain. 2nd ed. Edinburgh, Churchill Livingstone, 1989; with permission.)

Travell's and Simons' mapping (Fig. 7) of myofascial trigger points in each muscle provides the most detailed description of specific muscle reactions and reactions in functional muscular units. However, Janda's description of the patterns of muscular dysfunction is one of the most globally applicable:

> . . . development of tightness and/or weakness in certain muscles may be considered as a systemic and characteristic deviation in the functional quality of these muscles. The final result of this deviation is then a general imbalance with the whole muscular system.[19]

Systemic stress produces characteristic patterns in the lower and upper body (Table 1) that emphasizes the crossed nature of spasm in postural muscles and pseudoparesis in antagonist muscles. The hyperactive and inhibited muscles for each pattern are described in Table 1, and objective evidence for the cross-function of postural muscles is found in chapter 9. Selected individual muscles are discussed in the treatment section of this chapter. Clinicians should recognize from their own observations that dysfunction is commonly found in several of these muscles. Even experienced clinicians will enhance their clinical acumen by widening their perspective to recognize gravity as a systemic stressor and expanding their diagnostic examination to look for dysfunction in parts of the pattern not previously considered.

Soft tissue structures are affected early in patients with postural decompensation. Symptoms arising from the pathophysiology of soft tissues have certain palpable characteristics and general radiographic patterns. Postural alignment often directs the palpatory examination (Fig. 8). The palpatory examination should be designed to assess specifically the spinal transition areas, postural muscles and their

TABLE 1.   Muscle Response to Gravitational Strain

Postural Muscles	Phasic Muscles
Cervical/Upper Thoracic/Agonist/Antagonist	
Upper trapezius	Latissimus dorsi
Levator scapulae	
Pectoralis major (upper art)	Mid/lower trapezius
Pectoralis minor	Rhomboids
Cervical erector spinae	Anterior cervical muscles
Scalenus muscles	
Lumbar/Lumbopelvic/Agonist/Antagonist	
Tensor fasciae latae	
Hamstrings	Quadriceps
Hip adductors (short adductors)	
Gastrocnemius/soleus	Abdominals
Piriformis	
Iliopsoas	Gluteus maximus

antagonists, and ligamentous structures involved in the maintenance of postural alignment. Sclerotomal[16] and myotomal pain patterns should be recalled and elicited in the history. Weakness or muscle cramping, either isolated or in an apparent neurologic distribution, are also important in the assessment of the patient with postural decompensation. A neurologic examination and functional muscle testing are essential.

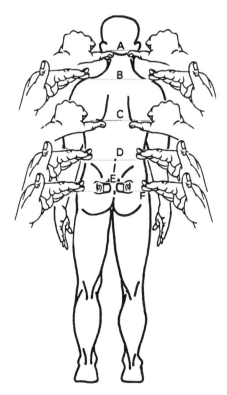

FIGURE 8.   After assessment of postural alignment in the sagittal plane (Fig. 1), postural alignment is assessed in coronal and horizontal planes. Observation typically precedes and directs the palpatory examination. A = occipital plane; B = shoulder plane; C = scapular plane (inferior); D = iliac crest plane; E = PSIS plane; F = greater trochanteric plane.

Levelness of Horizontal Planes

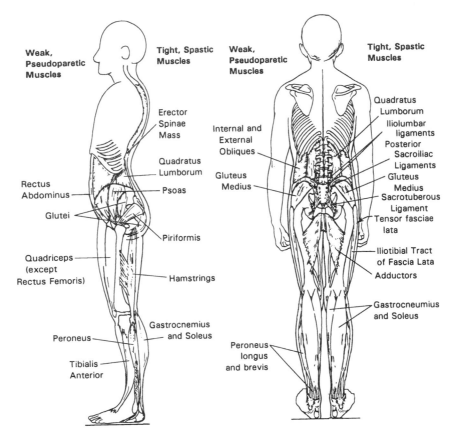

FIGURE 9. Significant postural and phasic muscles. Structures frequently stressed by gravity should be systematically palpated for spasm, trigger points, edema, or other evidence of dysfunction. In the presence of a pattern of structural dysfunction, gravitational strain pathophysiology should be considered as a primary etiologic factor.

Postural stress in the sagittal plane typically activates the systemic pattern described by Janda.[19] In addition, stress placed on ligamentous tissues results in sclerotomal and ligamentous pain patterns most obviously diagnosed by involvement of the iliolumbar ligaments bilaterally. Figure 9 illustrates the postural pattern and structures of the low back, pelvic girdle, and lower extremities that are strained by gravitational stress. Symptoms commonly referred from the musculoligamentous structures are delineated in Table 2. In these patients, the knees are often slightly flexed. Postural stress affecting the vastus medialis and lateralis leads to weakness in these muscles, with subsequent knee buckling and patellofemoral tracking problems. Patients complain of bilateral low back pain, which often takes more than 30 minutes to resolve even when they lie down and remove the longitudinal effect of gravity and easy fatigability. They also have a higher incidence of somatovisceral activation of functional disorders, such as irritable bowel syndrome or dysmenorrhea. Patients with high functional demand in the sagittal plane are more likely to develop hyperlordosis, spondylolysis, and isthmic L5–S1 spondylolisthesis.

TABLE 2.   Muscle Symptoms Arising From Gravitational Strain

Structure	Spastic Muscle Symptom
Iliopsoas	Inability to stand straight (psoas posturing); knees flexed; recurrent L1–2 somatic dysfunction; pain referral to back and anterior groin; positive Thomas test
Quadratus lumborum	Low back pain referred to the groin and hip; exhalation 12th rib somatic dysfunction; diaphragm restriction
Hamstrings	Pain sitting or walking; pain disturbs sleep; pain referral to posterior thighs; straight leg raising limited mechanically
Piriformis	Pain down posterior thigh; may entrap peroneal portion of sciatic nerve; perpetuated by sacroiliac dysfunction; associated with pelvic floor dysfunction, dyspareunia, and prostatodynia
Thigh adductors (short)	Pain referral to inguinal ligament, inner thigh, upper medial knee
Gastrocnemius-soleus complex	Nocturnal leg cramps; pain referral to upper posterior calf, instep, and heel

Structure	Inhibited Muscle Symptom
Gluteus minimus	Pain characteristic when arising from chair; pain referral to buttock, lateral and posterior thigh; "pseudosciatica"; antalgic gait; positive Trendelenburg test
Gluteus medius	Pain aggravated by walking; pain referral to posterior iliac rest and sacroiliac joint; positive Trendelenburg test
Gluteus maximus	Restlessness, pain sitting or walking up hill; antalgic gait
Vastus muscles	Buckling knee; weakness going up stairs; thigh and knee pain; chondromalacia patellae
Rectus abdominus	Increased lordosis; constipation
Tibialis anterior	Pain referred to great toe and anteromedial ankle; may drag foot or trip when tired

Postural stress in the coronal plane also contributes to the development of low back pain, which typically is accompanied by unilateral iliolumbar ligament strain and quadratus lumborum tightness. Postural curves in the coronal plane commonly include a single C-curve or the double S-type curve. Facilitated segments of the spinal cord are frequently associated with cross-over and apical spinal segments along these curves. Visceral organs obtaining their primary innervation from the facilitated cord segments often exhibit dysfunctional pathology associated with hypersympathetic activity. Regardless of the number of curves, musculoligamentous structures on the concave side of a curve are shortened, and those on the convex side are stretched. Typically postural stress in the horizontal plane accompanies that in the coronal plane.

RADIOGRAPHIC FINDINGS

A standardized radiographic study with the patient standing is the best method for determining the potential biomechanical consequences of variations in static postural alignment precisely. Many static postural measurements are associated with low back pain and other gravitational stress-induced clinical findings.[28] Objective and reproducible measurements outside normative ranges of a standardized protocol[42] (Fig. 10) suggest a biomechanical disadvantage that has been correlated with increased functional demand regionally. Through tensegrity principles, increased functional demand throughout the body is suggested. The larger the number of biomechanical risk factors and the greater degree of deviation from normative postural ranges, the more likely that homeostatic mechanisms for maintenance of posture

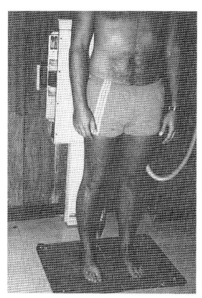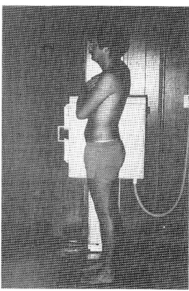

FIGURE 10. A radiographic protocol including a floor plate capable of being leveled perfectly in the horizontal plane and a plumb bob hung on a metallic wire to provide an absolute reference to the gravitational line when exposed onto the radiographic film assures accurate measurements. Standardization of patient foot and arm positions, including feet equidistant from the plumb bob and spaced under the hips, with locked knees, enhances reproducibility.

will fail. Biomechanical risk factors not only strain musculoligamentous structures but also predispose the patient to structural damage as in spondylolysis and/or spondylolisthesis.[7,30] Radiographs are also extremely valuable in identifying bony anomalies and other structural deficiencies that help functional stresses (such as gravity) to overwhelm the body's homeostatic mechanisms. The standardized protocol also demonstrates the effect of gravity on posture in a reproducible manner that permits objective documentation of response to treatment.

Key radiographic measurements are extracted from the standing lateral lumbopelvic radiograph. These measurements are easily and accurately determined by physicians.[35] Data then can be compared with normal ranges derived from the standardized radiographic protocol (Fig. 10). Radiographic measurements strongly correlate with one another and with dynamic findings. Comparison of postural measurements to normative ranges provides clinical insights for planning a management program.

One of these measurements, pelvic index (PI), is an infrequently reported but extremely valuable measurement for objective evaluation of intrapelvic gravitational strain. PI represents the relative position of the sacrum with respect to the innominate (pelvic) bones. An understanding of biomechanics (Fig. 11) readily suggests that PI objectively quantifies the accumulated pelvic effect of the battle between gravity and homeostatic mechanisms that help to resist it. This and other sagittal plane postural measurements may be followed over time to provide graphic, objective documentation of the patient's progress.

An anteroposterior (AP) lumbopelvic postural radiograph provides key measurements for the evaluation of postural alignment in the coronal and horizontal planes. It also provides an idea of the type and amount of postural compensation or

Halfsole
us heel lift !

PELVIC MECHANICS

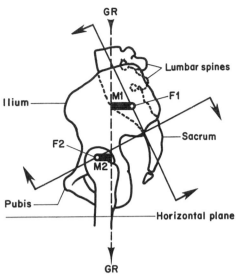

FIGURE 11. Intrapelvic rotations occur biomechanically about their axes of rotation (F1 and F2) in relation to the gravitational (GR) line.[21] The sacrum rotates anteriorly because weightbearing falls anterior to its S_2 axis. The innominates rotate posteriorly because weightbearing is posterior to the femoral axes.

the response to treatments that are designed to affect posture (Fig. 12). Variations of postural alignment and their relative frequency in the general population have been studied extensively (Fig. 13). Relationships between key structural landmarks are shown in Figure 14, and key postural measurements and their normative ranges are depicted in Figure 15. Such measurements may be followed to help determine the efficacy of treatment protocols in objective and graphic terms.

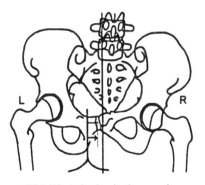

With lifts in heel or in the opposite half-sole, the pelvis can be derotated.

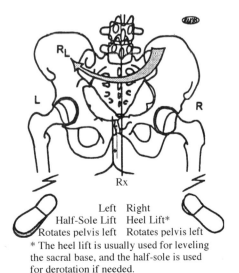

	Left	Right
	Half-Sole Lift	Heel Lift*
	Rotates pelvis left	Rotates pelvis left

* The heel lift is usually used for leveling the sacral base, and the half-sole is used for derotation if needed.

FIGURE 12. Sacral base unleveling and pelvic rotation are measured from the AP postural x-ray. The sacral base is extrapolated laterally to a point over each femoral head (see Fig. 14). This permits clinical determination of appropriate shoe lift therapy. Pelvic rotation is named for the direction in which the pubic symphysis moves relative to the gluteal cleft line.

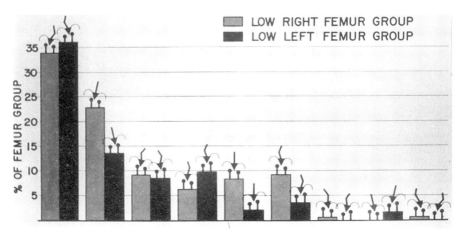

FIGURE 13.   Frequency distribution of mirror image patterns in low right and left femur groups (n = 738). This study from the Kirskville College of Osteopathic Medicine typifies postural alignment variations in the coronal plane.

SOMATIC DYSFUNCTION AND SEGMENTAL FACILITATION

Spinal somatic dysfunction is most prevalent at transitional areas of the spine. Characteristic findings include tenderness to palpation, asymmetry of position and motion, restriction to motion in a noncapsular pattern, and changes in tissue texture related to associated neural, vascular, and lymphatic dysfunction. Somatic dysfunction induced by gravitational stress is common. Chronic postural stress results in recurrent patterns of somatic dysfunction even after apparently successful treatment. Recurrent myofascial trigger point patterns are also a clue to chronic postural stress, strain, and decompensation.

Segmental and regional palpation of spinal motion characteristics, palpation of paraspinal tissues, and the discovery of somatic dysfunction provide information relevant to the dynamic aspects of posture. Numerous segmental and regional palpatory methods can provide this information. Segmental motion testing can be active or passive (see Fig. 15). Passive segmental motion testing is especially sensitive to characteristics or quality of the barrier to the minor, involuntary range of motion of a synovial joint. (Fig. 16). The characteristic feel of the barrier to passive motion is called *end-feel*. Mennell[38] described end-feel as loss of joint play, a small but precise amount of movement (less than $\frac{1}{8}$ inch) that is independent of voluntary muscle function. Loss of joint play results in a characteristic end-feel that is abrupt rather than resilient. Depending on the number of minor motions allowed by a joint structure, each synovial joint has one or more joint play movements that can be assessed. Passive motion testing and assessment of end-feel is the basis for diagnosis of joint somatic dysfunction. Each somatic dysfunction can be denoted specifically by describing its combination of motion restrictions.

Active segmental motion testing is performed by the patient, with the physician monitoring the outcome. Voluntary active motion at synovial joints depends on the integrity of joint play and the smooth action of the minor joint motions. In active motion testing of the spine, the physician palpates in the region of the articular facets and interprets motion characteristics as the patient bends backward and forward. Regardless of the type of motion testing, interexaminer reliability for de-

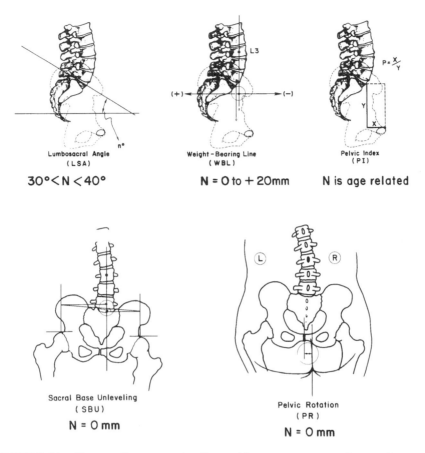

FIGURE 14. Key standing postural radiographic measurements and normative ranges. (From Kuchera WA, Kuchera ML: Osteopathic Principles in Practice. 2nd ed., revised. Columbus, OH, Greydon Press, 1994; with permission.)

termining segmental somatic dysfunction is high if the same diagnostic criteria are used.

Segmental somatic dysfunction may prevent the body from altering posture even when otherwise appropriate treatment protocols are offered. Although the precise mechanisms have not been isolated, the role of somatic dysfunction in central integration of proprioceptive and nociceptive input has been implicated. Others view somatic dysfunction as a mechanical deterrent to postural realignment. Regardless of the mechanism, correction of segmental somatic dysfunction plays an important role in restoration of joint play and the patient's ability to respond positively to postural treatment protocols.

In regional testing, the fascia associated with transition zones is moved in various directions and named for the direction in which the tissues move most freely. In compensatory fascial patterns, the direction in which the fascia prefers to move typically alternates at each transition zone.[43] Each sidebending curve to the right, for example, is balanced in the adjacent structural region by a sidebending curve to the left. Each region that prefers to rotate better to the right alternates with an adjacent

Passive

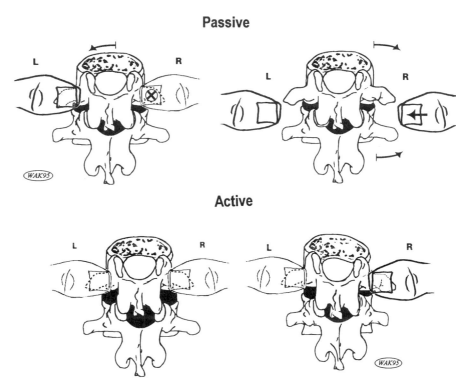

Active

FIGURE 15.   Motion testing. With passive motion testing (top), the patient is passive while the physician palpates the end-feel of the barriers of sidebending and rotation. In this case, the left thumb meets sudden resistance in both sidebending and rotation, and the right thumb meets a springing physiologic endpoint. Diagnosis: NS_RR_L. With active motion testing (bottom), the patient flexes (left) and extends (right) while the physician palpates the motion of the transverse processes. In this case, both thumbs move forward equally with flexion. With extension the right facet closes but the left does not. At the end of extension, the right transverse process is more posterior than the left. Diagnosis: F R_R S_R.

region preferring to rotate to the left. Thus, compensatory fascial patterns are balanced and alternating. Traumatically induced fascial patterns do not alternate and are less balanced or unbalanced (Fig. 17). Skeletal, arthrodial, and myofascial structures in transition areas also tend to move in the direction of fascial freedom. Thus, a fascial preference pattern determined by regional testing provides insight into the direction and amount of compensation in a biomechanically stressed patient. Correction of somatic dysfunction also is considered important to allow postural realignment and to prevent recurrent dysfunctional posture.

Afferent input from somatic dysfunction typically reports to related spinal levels at which segmental facilitation may be established. Segmental spinal cord facilitation is associated with lowered thresholds to somatic, visceral, and psychoemotional stressors and mediates somatosomatic, somatovisceral, viscerosomatic, and some viscerovisceral reflexes (Fig. 18). Travell and Simons[41] present a similar case to explain the characteristics of myofascial trigger points. Studies reveal that postural patterns can be mapped like fingerprints and are roughly recognizable years after initial documentation.[4] Likewise, if posture is modified experimentally by sys-

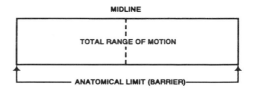

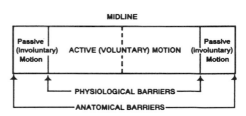

FIGURE 16. Physiologic, restrictive, and anatomic barriers. Each has a characteristic palpatory end-feel. (From Kuchera WA, Kuchera ML: Osteopathic Principles in Practice. 2nd ed., revised. Columbus, OH, Greydon Press, 1994; with permission.)

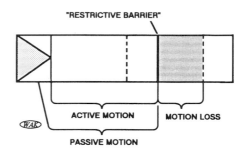

temic imbalance due to a nontherapeutic heel lift, patterns of somatic dysfunction and segmental facilitation are induced.

Thus, spinal somatic dysfunction induced by gravitational stress at postural cross-overs and other transition zones may create facilitated segments that function

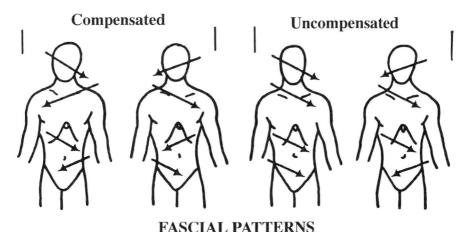

FIGURE 17. Compensated fascial patterns alternate. Typically, traumatically induced patterns do not alternate.

The Neurologic Lens

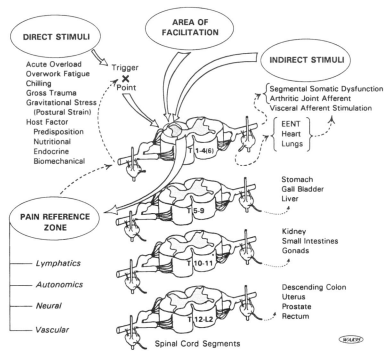

FIGURE 18.   Many direct stimuli are capable of initiating trigger points with distinct pain reference zones. Initiation is even more likely when indirect stimuli facilitate segmentally related levels. Conversely, trigger points are capable of facilitating the cord with somatic afferent stimuli. Resultant neural, lymphatic, and vascular changes affect segmentally related viscera. Feedback loops exist, creating somatosomatic, somatovisceral, viserosomatic, and viscerovisceral reflexes. The facilitated segment, therefore, plays a role in the maintenance of these reflexes and also acts as a "neurologic lens," enabling a variety of stressors to initiate both visceral and somatic symptoms. Bold arrows represent the main direction of neural communication. Dotted arrows represent feedback potential.

as a "neurologic lens,"[26] focusing stress on associated visceral and somatic structures. Treatment of postural disorders to promote better weightbearing alignment not only decreases musculoligamentous signs and symptoms but also provides a wide range of welcome and sometimes unexpected benefits for the patient.

TREATMENT PROTOCOLS TO RESTORE BIOMECHANICAL ALIGNMENT

The goal of treatment is to optimize biomechanical alignment and thus to maximize the structure-function interrelationships between gravitational stress and the patient. Treatment may include, but is not limited to, orthotics, manipulation, exercise protocols, physical therapy modalities, and, of course, patient education. Not all of these modalities are required in every patient, nor will every patient respond as hoped, even when the optimal combinations are applied. Treatment goals modalities are chosen (1) to significantly reduce symptoms, (2) to prevent permanent or struc-

tural change, (3) to arrest further decompensation in patients with struc'
and (4) occasionally to reverse a portion of the structural change.

Postural stress due to gravity manifests with several subjective sig
toms that may correlate with gross observation of posture, radiographic postura.
measurements, palpable diagnosis of recurrent arthrodial and myofascial dysfunctions, and localization of ligamentous strain. The remainder of this chapter discusses
aspects of treatment and presents protocols designed to meet the goals of treatment.

Orthotics—Coronal and Horizontal Planes

Lift therapy for coronal plane postural problems began to appear in medical literature in the mid nineteenth century and was specifically mentioned by John Hilton
in 1863:

> Thus I have seen many patients wearing spinal supports, in order to correct a lateral cur-
> vature when the deformity might have and has been subsequently, corrected by placing
> within the shoe or boot a piece of cork thick enough to compensate for the shortness of
> the less well developed limb.[15]

The osteopathic profession has thoroughly researched lift therapy protocols.
Articles published in the 1983 *Yearbook of the American Academy of Osteopathy*[39]
discuss the diagnosis, clinical impact, and treatment of coronal plane postural alignment. Travell and Simons emphasize the need for heel lifts for patients with inequality of leg lengths.[41] They also comment on the use of lifts for the ischial tuberosity in
patients with small hemipelvises to balance seated spinal posture. Balanced posture
eliminates one of the most common precipitating and/or perpetuating causes of myofascial trigger points. Numerous authors have shown that lift therapy reduces
chronic low back pain and has a significant effect on a number of somatic complaints affecting musculoligamentous structures.[9,18]

Patients with symptoms of musculoligamentous strain, sacral base unevenness,
and coronal plane postural imbalance due to gravitationally induced stresses may
benefit from a shoe lift on the side of the low sacral base. This is especially true if
the patient has a compensatory lumbar spinal curvature bent to the side opposite the
low sacral base. Typically, patients with acute back pain or patients with symptom
flare-up due to minimal aggravation are started on $1/16$" lift. Less fragile patients are
started with a $1/8$" lift. The lift can be increased by $1/16$" every 2 weeks or $1/8$" every
month. This progression tends to prevent musculoskeletal discomfort from too rapid
postural realignment.

Heilig reported attempts to formulate more specific guidelines to quantify the
initial amount of lift.[14] He found that an empirical formula was often inadequate or
too conservative. His formula considered the amount of lift to be directly proportional to the unevenness of the sacral base and inversely proportional to host factors
such as age, duration of the condition, and the amount of compensation or adaptation:

$$L < [SBU] / [D+C],$$

where L = initial lift required, SBU = sacral base unleveling, D = duration, and C =
compensation. Duration was further allotted as (1) = 0–10 years, (2) = 10–30 years,
and (3) = 30+ years. Compensation was categorized as (0) = none observed, (1) =
rotation of the lumbar vertebrae into the convexity of the compensatory sidebending, and (2) = wedging of the vertebrae, altered size of facets, horizontal osseous de-
velopments from the endplates, and/or spurring.

Occasionally the concavity of the spinal curve is toward the side of the short
lower extremity. In this less common situation, the physician first prescribes a lift

for the side of the long leg to change the lumbar scoliosis and relieve some of the pelvic and lumbar strain.[36] The lift on the long leg side is later reduced and the unlevel sacral base is lifted.

Except in highly sensitive patients, the heel usually can be lifted ½ inch without adding to the sole of the shoe. A higher lift produces significant pelvic rotation to the opposite side (see Fig. 12) and results in alteration of foot mechanics. When pelvic rotation to the side opposite the depressed sacral base should be beneficial, the heel lift also becomes therapeutic for postural alignment in the horizontal plane.

An anterior sole lift creates rotation to the same side as the lift and with less coronal plane adjustment than a heel lift. The anterior sole lift is used when significant ipsilateral rotation is needed to correct horizontal plane alignment. Clinically, horizontal rotation of less than 5 mm need not be treated. When pelvic rotation is 5–10 mm, sacral base unleveling should be treated with appropriate coronal plane principles, and the rotational component in the horizontal plane should be treated with an anterior lift, beginning with ⅛". The anterior lift is increased in ⅛-inch increments every 2 weeks. Pelvic rotation that exceeds 10 mm should be treated with inclusion of an initial anterior sole lift measuring ¼ inch. Combinations of heel and anterior lifts are increased according to principles discussed above for coronal and horizontal planes, respectively.

All shoe lift protocols involving anterior, heel, or entire sole lifts (Fig. 19) require concomitant use of manipulative treatment of somatic dysfunction, which

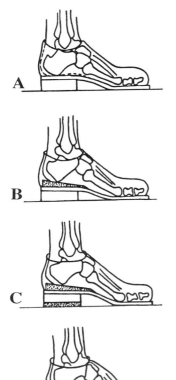

FIGURE 19. In general, lift therapy should begin with ¹⁄₁₆–⅛". A proportional rate of ⅙" per 2 weeks in increments of ¹⁄₁₆–⅛" permits time for the body to adjust. Lift therapy should always be accompanied by systemic manipulation and soft tissue stretching to permit optimal change with minimal side effects. *A*, foot in typical shoe. *B*, heel lift in place, amount of lift measured at midcalcaneal line. Maximum lift inside shoe is ¼". *C*, if more lift is needed, it can be added to the outside heel. Maximum lift under the heel (inside and/or outside) is ½". *D*, if more than ½" is needed, the entire sole must be lifted.

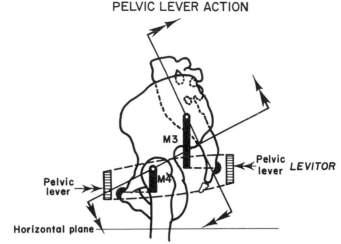

PELVIC LEVER ACTION

FIGURE 20. The leverage action of the Levitor[21] is accomplished through precise pad placement to resist gravitationally induced counterrotation of the sacrum and the innominates (Fig. 11). The anterior pad is placed on the anterosuperior aspect of the pubes; the sacral pad is placed below the S_2 axis.

allows comfortable adjustment and permits proper realignment. The patient's postural mechanisms should function within the parameters of the evolving new coronal and/or horizontal plane alignment; postural mechanisms are "reeducated" to this more ideal and biomechanically stable functional alignment. Paraspinal muscle tension becomes more symmetric. Clinically, symptoms throughout the body are reduced dramatically.

Orthotics—Sagittal Plane

Since most pelvic braces are static and designed for acute situations only, they are inadequate for treatment of chronic postural change. Only one pelvic orthotic, the Levitor, is both dynamic and designed to be worn for prolonged times in direct biomechanical opposition to the decompensating effect of gravitational strain in the sagittal plane (Fig. 20). Because it does not replace muscular action, prolonged use does not have the muscle-weakening side effect of static braces. The combination of a dynamic pelvic orthotic and the conservative postural protocol—manipulation, physical therapy, exercise, and patient education—is more effective than the conservative protocol by itself in the patients with chronic low back pain.[33]

The Levitor, which weighs 5–7 ounces, is constructed of a special aluminum alloy and is designed to transfer about 7 pounds of pressure to the pubic rami and the sacral base below the S2 pivot. This transfer induces counterrotation of the sacrum with respect to the innominates, reversing gravitationally induced musculoligamentous strain. In patients carefully selected to meet inclusion criteria set forth by the Institute for Gravitational Strain Pathology,[17] 86% experienced reduction of pain. In another study,[33] 76% of patients with difficult-to-manage low back pain demonstrated objective improvement of sagittal plane postural radiographic measurements compared with 33% of patients treated with physical therapy, manipulation, exercise, and patient education alone.

Pansystemic manipulation of somatic dysfunction is as vital to successful postural treatment in the sagittal plane as it is to postural alignment in coronal and/or horizontal planes. Hypomobility, in the presence of adaptive postural homeostatic mechanisms, disrupts the realignment process and creates the potential for new or aggravated pain from musculoligamentous strain.

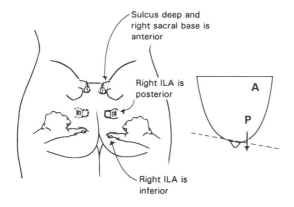

FIGURE 21. Palpatory findings of a right sacral shear include a deep right sulcus and a very inferior (and slightly posterior) inferolateral angle of the sacrum.

Labels in figure: Sulcus deep and right sacral base is anterior; Right ILA is posterior; A; P; Right ILA is inferior

Spinal and Extremity Joint Manipulation

In orthopedic medicine, manipulation is used in three distinct situations:[3]

1. To counter capsular contracture (stretching techniques);

2. To break down adhesive and fibrous connective tissues using (high-velocity, low-amplitude thrust or other direct manipulative techniques); and

3. To reestablish motion and alignment in joints with somatic dysfunction (wide range of manipulative techniques).

Manipulation is necessary for postural realignment when one needs to reestablish motion and alignment as well as break down shortened tissues. The choice of manipulative technique is much less important than accomplishing basic goals:

1. Restitution of lost normal motion;

2. Removal of central physiologic mechanisms that perpetuate somatic dysfunction; and

3. Modification of the physical impediments that block accomplishment of these goals.

Postural realignment and reduction of musculoligamentous strain requires that certain pelvic somatic dysfunctions be diagnosed and treated appropriately with manipulation, including three traumatically induced pelvic shear somatic dysfunctions: sacral shear, innominate shear, and pubic shear. Such shears often occur when patients unexpectedly step into a pot hole or off a step or curb that they did not anticipate. Force transferred up the lower extremity or into the ischial tuberosity is met by the downward force of the body's weight and momentum. The result is a shearing force along the sacroiliac articulation. The shape of the sacroiliac articulation influences the shearing movement of the sacroiliac, resulting in fairly predictable static palpatory landmarks along with restricted sacroiliac function (Fig. 21). Pubic shears also possess distinctive palpatory characteristics.

Although a number of manipulative techniques are described in the osteopathic literature[11, 24] to address sacroiliac shear, a straight longitudinal high-velocity, low-amplitude (HVLA) tug through the ipsilateral lower extremity is often successful. The soft tissue slack of the knee and hip is first eliminated with steady traction and encouragement of patients to relax their muscles. A HVLA tug is then applied against resistance applied to the sacrum. (Fig. 22). This technique is often effective in reestablishing both static alignment and dynamic motion in the sacroiliac joint.

Not all somatic dysfunction of the pelvis is due to traumatic shear; most occur during activities of daily living. Simply walking engages a number of physiologic axes, and momentary disruption of coordination during the walking cycle can result

Right Sacral Shear

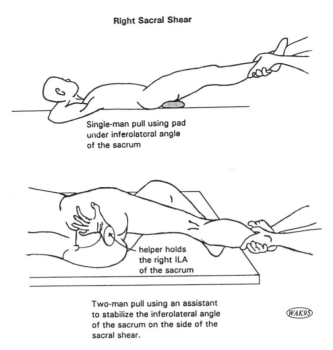

Single-man pull using pad
under inferolateral angle
of the sacrum

helper holds
the right ILA
of the sacrum

Two-man pull using an assistant
to stabilize the inferolateral angle
of the sacrum on the side of the
sacral shear.

WAK93

FIGURE 22. Manipulative treatment of a right sacral shear can be performed in a variety of ways: a single-operator direct method using a pad under the right inferolateral angle (ILA) of the sacrum (top), and a two-operator direct method using an assistant to stabilize the right sacral ILA (bottom).

in numerous types of somatic dysfunction involving the sacrum or innominates. Prolonged shifting of weight onto a potential axis of motion may engage it and predispose to somatic dysfunction around that axis. Golfers, for example, tend to develop a right rotation about a right oblique sacral axis, which may result from shifting weight onto the right upper pole of the sacrum during the golf swing. In the general population, the most common compensatory (nontraumatic) pattern of somatic dysfunction in the pelvis includes a left rotation about a left sacral oblique axis and an anteriorly rotated right innominate.

Innominate somatic dysfunction often responds well to muscle energy manipulative techniques designed to gap the sacroiliac joint. The dysfunctional barrier is engaged by rotating half of the pelvis in a manner that moves the static landmarks against the barrier. The patient is then asked to attempt to rotate the pelvis actively away from the impediment as the physician applies isometric resistance. When the patient is relaxed, the physician rotates the pelvis further through the dysfunctional barrier. This cycle is repeated about three times. If the innominate is rotated anteriorly or the pubic symphysis is inferior, the physician flexes the patient's knee and the thigh to position the lower extremity so that the hamstrings will pull (and rotate) the innominate posteriorly. If the innominate is rotated posteriorly or the pubic ramus is superior, the physician extends the patient's lower extremity to permit the quadriceps to pull (or rotate) the innominate anteriorly. In each of these positions, the physician positions the patient and holds the knee so that either activation pulls the origin of the muscles in the appropriate direction to correct the somatic dysfunc-

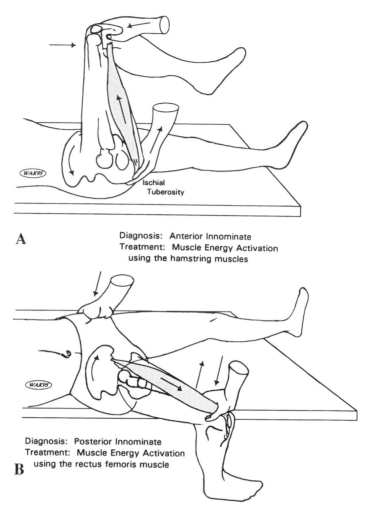

FIGURE 23. *A*, to treat a patient with the diagnosis of anterior innominate somatic dysfunction, a muscle energy direct method employs the hamstrings to rotate the innominate posteriorly through the restrictive barrier. *B*, to treat a patient with the diagnosis of posterior innominate somatic dysfunction, a muscle energy direct method employs the quadriceps to rotate the innominate anteriorly through the restrictive barrier.

tion (Fig. 23). The addition of sufficient adduction to gap sacroiliac dysfunction or abduction to gap pubic somatic dysfunction helps to localize such techniques for optimal effect.

Correction of psoas shortening is also vital in achieving postural realignment and reduction of musculoligamentous strain. Acute psoas spasm is characterized by tenderness of the iliacus point, as described by Jones.[20] It is successfully treated with a counterstrain manipulative technique designed to remove the spastic tendencies. In the supine position, the patient's legs and hips are bent to about 90°, with the foot of the involved side crossed over the opposite ankle. The hips externally rotate by letting the knees separate. This general position is modified with careful and precise positioning to relax the psoas muscle. The appropriate position is ascertained by at least an immediate 70% reduction in tenderness/pain to direct palpation of that psoas. Once located, the position is maintained for 90 seconds. This "position of ease" reduces noxious afferent stimuli conveyed to the spinal cord, and positioning of antagonist muscles reflexly relaxes the shortened spastic iliopsoas. The extremities are slowly and passively extended back onto the treatment table. Associated L1 or L2 dysfunction is almost always found with a shortened spastic psoas muscle and should be specifically addressed. Manipulative treatment to remove somatic dysfunction is essential to achieving and maintaining normal function of the iliopsoas muscle.

The manipulative technique selected to address somatic dysfunction is less important than the treatment goals. Options include stripping or transverse friction deep massage; myofascial spray-and-stretch with a vapocoolant spray; joint manipulation; and trigger point injections of soft tissues. Regardless of the technique, manipulation of the afferent musculoskeletal input with respect to the central nervous system remains an essential element in all treatment protocols described in this chapter. Manipulation alone, however, provides only transient relief; somatic dysfunction recurs in predictable patterns and makes the patient dependent on manipulative procedures. If Lewit's perception that the most frequent cause of somatic dysfunction is faulty movement patterns potentiated by muscle imbalance and postural overstrain[37] is valid, clinicians treating patients with somatic dysfunction must consider a role for muscular reeducation and postural balancing.

Muscular Re-education

The central nervous system functions to coordinate patterns of movement rather than to activate isolated muscles. Movement precedes postural control and is necessary to alter it.[25] Thus, postural realignment cannot occur without muscular reeducation. Conversely, reestablishment of normal muscle function and central nervous system regulation of movement patterns depends on postural realignment. Coordinated, functional movement patterns and postural realignment are therefore interdependent.

The clinical goal is to return the patient with gravitational stress-induced musculoligamentous strain to normal function. Addressing the interdependence of postural stability, consistent proprioceptive input, and coordinated movement patterns requires a carefully constructed program and patient education. As in the selection of manipulation, a wide range of therapeutic techniques are available to reestablish normal movement patterns within the gravitational field. Certain principles, however, facilitate this goal regardless of the technique used:

1. **Seek biomechanical stability**. Biomechanical stability provides a balanced platform from which to operate. If orthotics are required, they should be worn consistently when the patient is in the upright position, especially early in the reeducation period when the central nervous system is integrating the evolving postural alignment.

2. **Stretch tight postural muscles or other shortened muscles**. Tight muscles should be stretched before attempting to strengthen inhibited, weakened muscles. Attempts to reverse this order are typically frustrating because inhibition from the shortened antagonist interferes with programs designed to strengthen the weakened phasic muscles.

3. **Keep functional units in careful balance with one another through proprioceptive retraining**. Such balance, which greatly facilitates treatment and fore-

stalls recurrence of dysfunction, can be achieved with a tilt board, by balancing on a large ball, or through a combination of specific exercises, as described by Janda.[19]

Prolotherapy for Hypermobile Regions

Not all hypermobile areas are structurally hypermobile; functional or compensatory hypermobility occurs as an early response to adjacent areas of hypomobile somatic dysfunction. Compensatory hypermobility disappears when the somatic dysfunction is removed. Over time, however, compensatory hypermobility adapts structurally to the constant functional demand, resulting in permanent or viscous change of musculoligamentous structures. Likewise, continuous gravitational stress may induce structural change at fibroosseous junctions and create structurally hypermobile areas. This "ligamentous relaxation" is responsible for continued chronic and recurrent pain in the neck and low back.[12] Further postural stress on hypermobile structures results in further discomfort, typically in the patterns described above. Patients cannot sit or stand in the gravitational field, even for short times, because they are unable to find a comfortable position. This condition is sometimes referred to as the "cocktail party syndrome."[5] Ligamentous relaxation affects tensegrity and therefore influences structures that may be quite distant from the locally hypermobile site.

In an attempt to protect joint structures, the body responds to hypermobility by depositing calcium along lines of stress. This response is often demonstrated radiographically as ligament calcification or bony exostoses. The iliolumbar ligament displays this phenomenon early in the process because its purpose is to stabilize the lumbar spine with respect to the pelvis and thus to permit postural function in the gravitational field (see Fig. 6).

The presence of structural hypermobility should alert the physician to the fact the affected areas are stressed beyond their homeostatic capabilities and need increased stability. Stability sometimes can be increased with conservative protocols that strengthen muscle and supplement the function of weakened ligaments. Proliferent therapy, or prolotherapy, also may eliminate structural hypermobility and is the treatment of choice for other patients with ligamentous laxity. As with all postural treatment protocols, if prolotherapy is improperly applied without addressing the alignment and motion aspects of the underlying gravitational stress problem, the clinical results will be unsatisfactory.

SUMMARY

Obviously, one solution for ligamentous relaxation and other structural decompensation is prevention. The success of this approach is enhanced by early identification of patients with biomechanical risk factors and recognition of symptoms associated with strain. The goal of prevention is to reduce risk factors and strengthen host factors before structural changes in the ligaments are permanent.

Prevention is not always possible. Recognition of the pathophysiologic mechanisms involved in gravitational stress and postural compensation/decompensation offers significant clinical insight into patient management. Biomechanical alignment and function are more likely to be restored and maintained if the physician offers a balanced total treatment protocol rather than a series of therapeutic interventions. Restoration of normal joint and regional stability improves biomechanical resistance to gravitational strain and postural decompensation. Correction of structural hypermobility improves the ability to resist gravitational stress-induced exaggeration of postural curves. Functional biomechanical aspects of the total treatment protocol are therefore more likely to be maintained by stabilizing structure. Somatic dysfunction is less likely to recur, and recurrent episodes are more easily treated with manipulative techniques. Muscular reeducation and restoration of muscle balance are also more easily accomplished.

REFERENCES

1. Beal MC: Biomechanics: A foundation for osteopathic theory and practice. In Northup GW (ed): Osteopathic Research: Growth and Development. Chicago, AOA Press, 1987, pp 37–57.
2. Cantu RI, Grodin AJ: Myofascial Manipulation: Theory and Clinical Application. Gaithersburg MD, Aspen, 1992.
3. Cyriax JH, Cyriax PJ: Cyriax's Illustrated Manual of Orthopaedic Medicine. 2nd ed. Oxford, Butterworth-Heinemann, 1993.
4. Denslow JS, Chace JA: Mechanical stresses in the human lumbar spine and pelvis (1962). In Beal M (ed): 1993 American Academy of Osteopathy Yearbook: Selected Papers of John Stedman Denslow, DO. Indianapolis, American Academy of Osteopathy, 1993.
5. Dorman TA, Ravin TH: Diagnosis and Injection Techniques in Orthopedic Medicine. Baltimore, Williams & Wilkins, 1991.
6. Dunnington WP: A musculoskeletal stress pattern: Observations from over 50 years' clinical experience. J Am Osteopath Assoc 64:366–371, 1964.
7. Educational Council on Osteopathic Principles: Glossary of osteopathic terminology. In 1995 AOA Yearbook and Directory of Osteopathic Physicians. 86th ed. Chicago, American Osteopathic Association, 1995.
8. Freeman JT: Posture in the aging body. JAMA 165:843–846, 1957.
9. Friberg O: Clinical symptoms and biomechanics of lumbar spine and hip joint in leg length inequality. Spine 8:643–651, 1983.
10. Gossman MR, Sahrmann SA, Rose SJ: Review of length-associated changes in muscle. Phys Ther 62:1799–1807, 1982.
11. Greenman PE: Principles of Manual Medicine. Baltimore, Williams & Wilkins, 1989.
12. Hackett GS: Low back pain. Ind Med Surg 28:416–419, 1959.
13. Hackett GS: Ligament and Tendon Relaxation Treated by Prolotherapy. 3rd ed. Springfield, IL, Charles C. Thomas, 1958.
14. Heilig D: Principles of lift therapy. In Peterson B (ed): Postural Balance and Imbalance. Newark OH, American Academy of Osteopathy, 1983, pp 113–118.
15. Hilton J: Rest and Pain. 6th ed. Philadelphia, JB Lippincott, 1950.
16. Inman VT, Saunders JB: Referred pain from skeletal structures. J Nerv Ment Dis 99:660–667, 1959.
17. Institute for Gravitational Strain Pathology: The Jungmann Concept and Technique of Antigravity Leverage. 2nd ed. Rangeley ME, Institute for Gravitational Strain Pathology, 1992.
18. Irvin RE: Reduction of lumbar scoliosis by use of a heel lift to level the sacral base. J Am Osteopath Assoc 91: 34–44, 1991.
19. Janda V: Muscle weakness and inhibition (pseudoparesis) in back pain syndromes. In Grieve GP (ed): Modern Manual Therapy of the Vertebral Column. Edinburgh, Churchill Livingstone, 1986, pp 197–200.
20. Jones L: Strain and Counterstrain. Indianapolis, American Academy of Osteopathy, 1993.
21. Jungmann M, McClure CW: Backaches, postural decline, aging and gravity-strain. Presented at the New York Academy of General Practice, New York, October 17, 1963.
22. Kapandji IA: Physiology of the Joints. Vol 3. New York, Churchill Livingstone, 1974.
23. Kendall FP, McCreary EK, Provance PG: Muscles: Testing and Function, with Posture and Pain. 4th ed. Baltimore, Williams & Wilkins, 1993.
24. Kimberly P (ed): Outline of Osteopathic Manipulative Procedure. 93rd ed. Kirksville MO, KCOM Press, 1980.
25. Knott M, Voss DE: Proprioceptive Neuromuscular Facilitation: Patterns and Techniques. 2nd ed. New York, Harper & Row, 1968.
26. Korr IM: The neural basis of the osteopathic lesion. J Am Osteopath Assoc 47:191–198, 1947.
27. Kuchera ML: Conservative management of symptomatic spondylolisthesis [FAAO thesis]. Indianapolis, American Academy of Osteopathy, 1986.
28. Kuchera ML: Gravitational strain pathophysiology: Parts I & II. In Vleeming A (ed): Low Back Pain: The Integrated Function of the Lumbar Spine and Sacroiliac Joints (in press).
29. Kuchera ML: Gravitational strain pathophysiology and "Unterkreuz" syndrome. Manuelle Medizin 33(2):56, 1995.

30. Kuchera ML: Postural decompensation in isthmic L5–S1 spondylolisthesis. J Am Osteopath Assoc 87:781, 1987.
31. Kuchera ML: Travell myofascial trigger points. In Ward R (ed): Foundations of Osteopathic Medicine. Williams & Wilkins (in press).
32. Kuchera ML, Irvin RE: Biomechanical considerations in postural realignment. J Am Osteopath Assoc 87:781–782, 1987.
33. Kuchera ML, Jungmann M: Inclusion of Levitor Orthotic Device in the management of refractive low back pain patients. J Am Osteopath Assoc 86: 673, 1986.
34. Kuchera ML, Kuchera WA: Osteopathic Considerations in Systemic Dysfunction. 2nd ed. Columbus OH, Greyden Press, 1994.
35. Kuchera ML, Bemben MG, Kuchera WA, Willman M: Comparison of manual and computerized methods of assessing postural radiographs. J Am Osteopath Assoc 90:714–715, 1990.
36. Kuchera WA, Kuchera ML: Osteopathic Principles in Practice. 2nd ed. Columbus OH, Greyden Press, 1994.
37. Lewit K: Manipulative Therapy in Rehabilitation of the Motor System. London, Butterworth, 1985.
38. Mennell J: Joint Pain: Diagnosis and Treatment using Manipulative Techniques. Boston, Little, Brown & Co, 1964.
39. Peterson B (ed): Postural Balance and Imbalance. 1983 Yearbook of the American Academy of Osteopathy. Newark OH, American Academy of Osteopathy, 1983.
40. Travell JG, Simons DG: Myofascial Pain and Dysfunction: The Trigger Point Manual. Vol 1. Baltimore, Williams & Wilkins, 1983.
41. Travell JG, Simons DG: Myofascial Pain and Dysfunction: The Trigger Point Manual. Vol 2. Baltimore, Williams & Wilkins, 1992.
42. Willman MK: Radiographic technical aspects of the postural study (1977). In Peterson B (ed): Postural Balance and Imbalance. Newark OH, 1983 Yearbook of the American Academy of Osteopathy , 1983, pp 140–143.
43. Zink JG, Lawson WB: An osteopathic structural examination and functional interpretation of the soma. Osteopath Ann 7:12–19, 1979.

RICHARD L. DONTIGNY, PT

FUNCTIONAL BIOMECHANICS AND MANAGEMENT OF PATHOMECHANICS OF THE SACROILIAC JOINTS

From DonTigny Physical Therapy
Havre, Montana

Reprint requests to:
Richard L. DonTigny, PT
P.O. Box 2514
115 Second Street West
Havre, MT 59501

To manage the pathomechanics of dysfunction of the sacroiliac joints effectively, it is necessary to understand the mechanics of normal function. An exercise program must be designed to restore and maintain normal function and to prevent the recurrence of dysfunction. Because the intervertebral disk is widely assumed to be the cause of most low back pain and because much low back pain is associated with postures that increase intradiskal pressure, many back school programs were developed to minimize intradiskal pressure. These programs persist despite the lack of demonstrated efficacy.[26]

Increases in intradiskal pressure, as measured by Nachemson,[29] are normal. They cause the nucleus to push against and stiffen the annulus and thus allow increased weight-loading. Although excessive compression may rupture the vertebral endplate, resulting in a Schmorl's node, the annulus does not tend to fail with compressive loading but rather as a result of shear loading.[19]

McKenzie advocated eccentric loading of the spine posteriorly to force the nucleus to move anteriorly and the annulus to bulge anteriorly.[27] Although occasionally effective, this method has a low intertester reliability, probably because several researchers have found that with eccentric loading the annulus always bulges on the loaded side and stiffens on the side under tension.[4,6,20,24,34,35,44]

Despite the apparent complexity of the problem, White made the following suggestion:

SPINE: State of the Art Reviews—Vol. 9, No. 2, May 1995
Philadelphia, Hanley & Belfus, Inc.

491

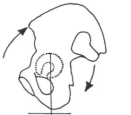 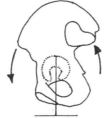

FIGURE 1. The innominate bones rotate anteriorly and posteriorly on an acetabular axis, raising and lowering the sacrum but not necessarily moving on the sacrum.

> It may well be that idiopathic backache will be found to be caused by some condition that is a subtle variation from normal. Otherwise, we probably would have found the cause already. If back pain were caused by a highly unusual condition, then fewer people would suffer from this disorder.[45]

Shaw's study of 2,000 consecutive cases of low back pain found that 98% had a dysfunction of the sacroiliac joints,[36] indicating that this subtle variation from normal may be found in the pathomechanics of the sacroiliac joints. Because the sacroiliac joints are structurally so strong and normal movement is so slight as to be nearly nonexistent, these joints have been assumed to be immune to injury through minor trauma and are seldom included in assessments of low back pain. This chapter describes the function of the sacroiliac joints; a specific, measurable, reversible, biomechanical dysfunction of the sacroiliac joint; and management of this dysfunction.

BIOMECHANICS AND FUNCTION

Movement

Movements of the innominate bones and the sacrum are only somewhat interdependent. The innominate bones rotate anteriorly and posteriorly on an acetabular axis (Fig. 1). Although this movement may raise or lower the sacrum, it does not necessarily cause movement in the sacroiliac joints. The sacroiliac joints tend to move with flexion (nutation) and extension (contranutation) of the spine (Fig. 2), although in fact movement may not occur.

Angulation of the joint surfaces is such that if movement of the sacrum were unrestricted by ligaments, the superincumbent weight would cause the S1 segment of the sacral surface of the sacroiliac joint to move downward and to separate from the S1 segment of the ilial surface (Fig. 3). Similarly, the S3 segment of the sacral

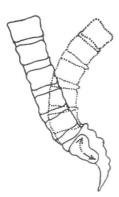

FIGURE 2. Any tendency toward movement of the sacrum on the ilial surface of the sacroiliac joint occurs with flexion and extension of the spine. Movement would tend to take place on a transverse axis, probably through the posterior aspect of the joint.

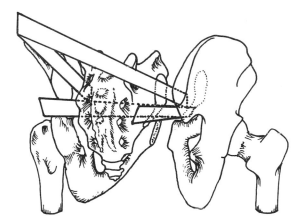

FIGURE 3.   Angulation of the joint surfaces.

surface of the sacroiliac joint would tend to rise and separate from the S3 segment of the ilial surface. Ligamentous restrictions, however, cause the sacroiliac joints to function in a unique manner.

Ligamentous Influence

The sacrum is slung from the posterosuperior iliac spines by the dense posterior interosseus ligaments. When the body moves from recumbency to an erect pos-

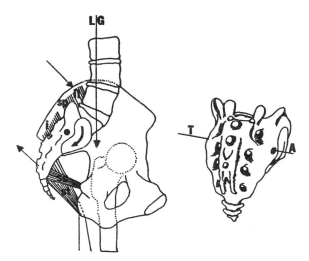

FIGURE 4.   Ligamentous tensile stress at the sacroiliac joint on a stabilized pelvis, independent of the ground reaction force vector through the acetabular axis. As the superincumbent weight through the line of gravity (LG) places a gravitational tensile stress on the posterior interosseus ligament (i), the short posterior sacroiliac ligament (sp), and the iliolumbar ligament (il) that results in a countergravitational stress on the sacrotuberous (st) and sacrospinous (ss) ligaments. The countergravitation stress creates a force-couple and causes a force-dependent transverse axis perpendicular to the opposing tensile forces. (From DonTigny RL: Function of the lumbosacroiliac complex as self-compensating force couple with a variable, force-dependent transverse axis: A theoretical analysis. J Man Manip Ther 2:87–93, 1994; with permission.)

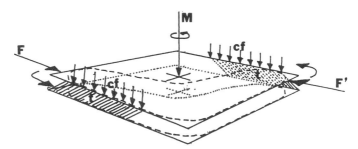

FIGURE 5. As the forces F and F' tend to rotate the superior structure around a force dependent axis (M), the rotational force creates a tensile stress on the tethering ligamentous attachment to the lower structure (t) and results in a compressive force (cf) between them. If the angle of the force at F or F' is changed, the location of the axis will be changed. If these forces are reversed, compression is decreased. Without the application of forces F and F' there can be no transverse axis of rotation. (From DonTigny RL: Function of the lumbosacroiliac complex as self-compensating force couple with a variable, force-dependent transverse axis: A theoretical analysis. J Man Manip Ther 2:87–93, 1994; with permission.)

ture, the superincumbent weight is transferred from the sacrum to the ilia through the posterior interosseus ligaments. The transfer of weight has three major effects: (1) approximation of the posterosuperior iliac spines, (2) slight caudal gliding of the sacral surface of the sacroiliac joint on the ilial surface, and (3) tensing of the sacrotuberous ligament. The tensile stress on the posterior interosseus and sacrotuberous ligaments is a force-couple acting on the sacrum and results in a moment that serves as a force-dependent axis of rotation for the sacroiliac joints[17] (Fig. 4).

Tensile stress also approximates the joint surfaces, and the increase in friction and stability causes a self-bracing of each joint (Fig. 5). Posterior rotation of the innominate bones on the acetabular axis increases the tensile force on the sacrotuberous ligament and hence the self-bracing. Self-bracing is probably most stable at the S1 segment of the sacroiliac joint for two reasons: (1) it begins at the S1 segment and proceeds sequentially to the S3 segment, and (2) the posterior interosseus ligaments are relatively short and dense. Anterior rotation of the innominate bone on the sacrum decreases tension on the sacrotuberous ligament and releases self-bracing first at the S3 segment. This arrangement allows increased joint stability and storage and release of energy in the ligaments without excessive compression of the joints.

During normal gait the trunk accelerates anteriorly, decelerates with impact-loading on the ipsilateral leg and then recovers to help propel the contralateral leg

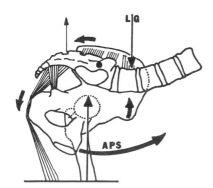

FIGURE 6. In forward flexion of the trunk, the line of gravity (LG) is anterior to the acetabula and creates a tendency for the innominate bones to rotate anteriorly. This must be countered by strong anterior pelvic support (APS) to maintain self-bracing and to balance forces through the lumbosacroiliac complex. (From DonTigny RL: Function of the lumbosacroiliac complex as self-compensating force couple with a variable, force-dependent transverse axis: A theoretical analysis. J Man Manip Ther 2:87–93, 1994; with permission.)

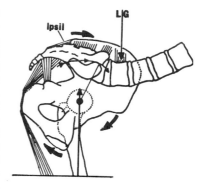

FIGURE 7. Lack of anterior pelvic support allows the innominate bones to rotate anteriorly on an acetabular axis, loosening the sacrotuberous and sacrospinous ligaments and decreasing self-bracing and friction. The innominate bone(s) shears cephalad and laterally on the sacrum at the posteroinferior iliac spine and downward anteriorly at the S1 segment. The rapid release of balanced force in this complex may cause a sudden stress on the paravertebral extensors, hamstrings, piriformis, and other related structures. The superficial long posterior sacroiliac ligaments (lpsil) are particularly vulnerable. (From DonTigny RL: Function of the lumbosacroiliac complex as self-compensating force couple with a variable, force-dependent transverse axis: A theoretical analysis. J Man Manip Ther 2:87–93, 1994; with permission.)

forward for the next step.[14,39] This rhythmic sacrocranial vertebral oscillation is controlled and damped by alternate self-bracing and release of each sacroiliac joint. When the body leans forward to perform any task, such as lifting, bending, or lowering, that may cause both innominate bones to rotate anteriorly on an acetabular axis, tightening of the abdominal muscles and strong support of the anterior pelvis are necessary to maintain the self-bracing bilaterally[17] (Fig. 6).

PATHOMECHANICS

Anterior rotation of the innominate bones around an acetabular axis without support of the anterior pelvis decreases tension on the sacrotuberous and sacrospinous ligaments and allows a decrease of self-bracing and friction bilaterally. As a result, instead of a tendency to movement of the sacral surface on the ilium on a transverse or oblique axis through the sacroiliac joints, the ilial surface of the sacroiliac joint may move on the sacral surface on an acetabular axis[13–15,17] (Fig. 7). A measurable movement of the posterosuperior iliac spines cephalad and laterally on the sacrum[16] stretches the superficial long posterior sacroiliac ligaments[42] and

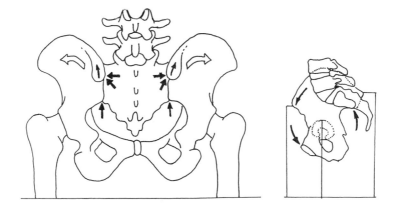

FIGURE 8. Posterior and lateral views of a bilateral anterior dysfunction. (From DonTigny RL: Mechanics and treatment of the sacroiliac joint. J Man Manip Ther 1:3–12, 1993; with permission.)

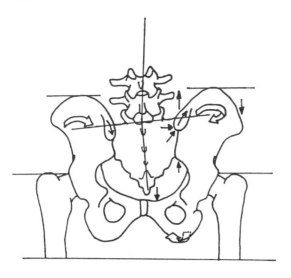

FIGURE 9. Posterior view of a right anterior dysfunction with the patient standing. (From DonTigny RL: Mechanics and treatment of the sacroiliac joint. J Man Manip Ther 1:3–12, 1993; with permission.)

causes pain along the lateral border of the sacrum. Tearing of this ligament may result in joint instability.

As the posterior aspects of the iliac crests rotate anteriorly, the tension on the iliolumbar ligaments may be decreased. Thus lumbosacral stability is also decreased, whereas the anterior inclination of the sacral plateau is increased. The end result is increased shear forces on the disks, increased stress on a spondylolisthesis, or an unstable lumbosacral segment. If damping of local oscillation or vibration is impaired, a vibrational tissue creep may increase instability and shear. As the innominate bone(s) rotate on the acetabular axis, the anterior capsule of the sacroiliac joint may be stretched or torn. Synovial fluid may leak from the joint and irritate the lumbosacral plexus and other sensitive structures nearby. Separation of the fibers of the iliacus at its conjoint origin with the sacrum may cause pain in the hip flexors. The flexors may appear to be dysfunctional when in fact the problem is dysfunctional anterior rotation. The pelvis may be inclined anteriorly, stretching the iliopsoas and giving the impression of tight hip flexors. Any attempt to stretch the hip flexors in such patients increases the anterior dysfunction of the sacroiliac joints and hence the pain.

In addition, cephalic shearing of the posterior ilia may stretch or tear the joint capsule of the S3 segment at the dorsal horn, deep to the conjoint origin of the gluteus maximus muscle in the area of the posteroinferior iliac spine. Depending on the extent and severity of the dysfunction, the fibers of the gluteus maximus may be separated on a line from its conjoint origin to the greater trochanter. The clinical complaint may be mistaken for piriformis pain; however, the body of the piriformis originates lower on the anterior surface of the sacrum. Separation of the fibers may cause pain around the trochanter and initiate bursitis with subsequent pain down the iliotibial band. The gluteus maximus may become swollen and congested in this area, and the point of pain at the posteroinferior iliac spine is not immediately obvious until the area is decongested by massage.

In patients with bilateral dysfunction, as the innominate bones rotate anteriorly on an acetabular axis, the sacroiliac joints are lifted and rise above the acetabula, causing an apparent change in the height of the posterosuperior iliac spines and the iliac crest when the patient is standing or an apparent lengthening of the legs when the patient is supine (Fig. 8). If the dysfunction is unilateral or asymmetrical, the

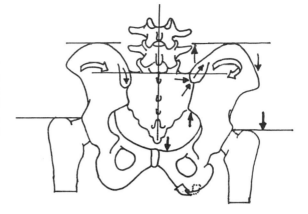

FIGURE 10. Posterior view of a right anterior dysfunction with the patient supine. (From DonTigny RL: Mechanics and treatment of the sacroiliac joint. J Man Manip Ther 1:3–12, 1993; with permission.)

crest on the affected side will be higher when the patient is standing (Fig. 9), and the leg on the affected side will appear to be longer when the patient is supine (Fig. 10), if one compares the relative length of each leg at the malleoli. The posterosuperior iliac spine will be higher on the more painful side when the patient is standing, and the sacral plateau will tilt away from the side of pain. Any resultant lateral shift will be away from the side of pain, and a compensatory scoliosis may occur toward the painful side when the patient is standing. As the innominate bone on the more painful side rises and moves somewhat anteriorly to the ipsilateral acetabula (or the

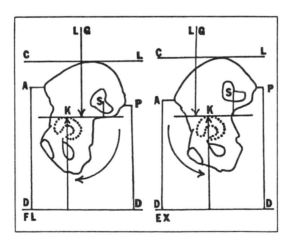

FIGURE 11. In the flexion position (FL), the line of gravity (LG) is posterior to the acetabula and causes a posterior rotational force around the acetabula. As the line of gravity moves anteriorly to the acetabula in the extension position (EX), the pelvis rotates anteriorly around the acetabula. The top of the acetabula (K) to the base (DD) remains constant. Although the height of the posterosuperior iliac spine (PD) and of the anterosuperior iliac spine (AD) changes considerably, the level of the crests of the ilia (CL) may not change significantly. As the level of the sacroiliac joint (S) rises, apparent leg length is increased in both supine and standing positions. The horizontal distance from K to S becomes shorter; thus, in the patient with sacroiliac joint dysfunction, leg length may be shorter during sitting but longer when positioned supine. (From DonTigny RL: Sacroiliac joint dysfunction [independent-study course]. Berryville, VA, Forum Medicum, Inc., 1990; with permission.)

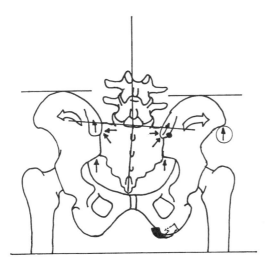

FIGURE 12. Posterior view of a bilateral anterior dysfunction compromised right, standing. (From DonTigny RL: Mechanics and treatment of the sacroiliac joint. J Man Manip Ther 1:3–12, 1993; with permission.)

acetabula moves posteriorly and caudad to the sacroiliac joint), the leg on the affected side will appear to be shorter in the long-sitting position (Fig. 11).

An apparent complication of simple bilateral anterior dysfunction is secondary vertical shifting of the S1 segment. The cephalad and lateral movement of the posterosuperior iliac spines on the sacrum slightly opens the sacroiliac joints, decreasing contiguity and friction in the anterior aspect of the joint. As a result, the anterior aspect of the innominate surface of the sacroiliac joint may slip vertically upward on the anterior aspect of the sacral surface if the innominate bone rotates posteriorly in an attempt to reestablish self-bracing. The initial point of binding appears to become a pathologic axis of rotation that allows the secondary shifting. This secondary shift may occur suddenly with initial impact during walking, causing the patient to collapse without warning. Dorman termed this phenomenon "the slipping clutch syndrome."[18] It is also referred to as an upslip or as a posterior innominate and frequently is mistaken for an anterior dysfunction on one side and a posterior dysfunction on the other. The iliac crest will be slightly lower on the more painful side

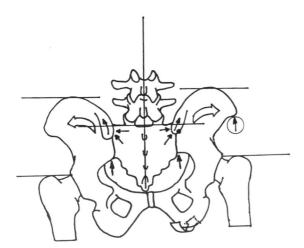

FIGURE 13. Posterior view of a bilateral anterior dysfunction compromised right, supine. (From DonTigny RL: Mechanics and treatment of the sacroiliac joint. J Man Manip Ther 1:3–12, 1993; with permission.)

when the patient is standing, and the leg on the more painful side will appear to be shorter when the patient is supine (Figs. 12 and 13). The posterosuperior iliac spine will be lower on the more painful side when the patient is standing, and the sacral plateau will tilt toward the same side. Any resultant lateral shift will be toward the more painful side when the patient is standing, and a compensatory scoliosis may develop away from the painful side.[15]

Caudally, as the ischial tuberosities approximate the coccyx, tension is decreased in the sacrotuberous ligaments and probably in the muscles and fascia of the pelvic diaphragm. This process may decrease sphincter control. If the tissues are allowed to remain in a shortened position, they may undergo a functional shortening that precludes restoration of the normal function of the lumbosacroiliac complex.

The decrease in self-bracing and decreased tension in the sacrotuberous ligament result in overuse in the biceps femoris, which may be an attempt to stabilize the sacrum through the sacrotuberous ligament. The patient may have an associated tendinitis in the tendon of the biceps femoris, posterior to the ischial tuberosity, and the ligaments of the head of the fibula may be strained by abnormal stress from the biceps femoris. This stress may continue distally and cause pain in the peroneus longus. Vleeming found that the peroneus longus may provide up to 40% of the stability of the sacrotuberous ligament through the kinetic chain.[43]

Pain and some displacement may occur at the pubic symphysis from abnormal torsion and stress.[12] Low back pain from an anterior rotation dysfunction of the sacroiliac joints may be increased with coughing, sneezing, or straining, because the rise in intraabdominal pressure tends to spread and flare the innominate bones. Pain may be referred into the groin and testicles and result in pseudoepididymitis. Pain in the abdomen at Baer's point varies with stress on the sacroiliac joint and may be misdiagnosed as appendicitis or ovarian pain. Baer's point is located 2 inches from the umbilicus on a line from the umbilicus to the anterosuperior iliac spine.[3,28] Wilson warned that radiation from the lower lumbar joints has led to unnecessary removal of pelvic organs.[46] Norman injected the sacroiliac joints and relieved the lower abdominal pain.[30] This pain also may be relieved by manual correction of the dysfunction.

Grieve found that sacroiliac strains sometimes follow gynecologic and obstetric operations.[21] Hormonal ligamentous laxity occurs during the last trimester of pregnancy[7,9] and to a lesser degree during menstruation and menopause.[9] Postmortem specimens in various stages of pregnancy clearly showed that the increased range of movement is easily recognizable by the fourth month and that at full term the range increased by about 2.5 times the normal value. In one subject, the anterior margins of the joint could be separated by almost 2 cm.[5] Movement abnormalities of the sacroiliac joints and pubic joints are a common cause of persistent postpartum pain, and simple mobilizing techniques localized to the sacroiliac joints are effective in alleviating such pain.[22] Davis and Lentle used technetium-99m stanous pyrophosphate bone scanning with quantitative sacroiliac scintigraphy in 50 female patients with idiopathic low back pain syndrome (age range = 21–71 years; mean = 39 years) and found that 22 patients (44%) had sacroiliitis. Eight of the 22 patients (36%) had unilateral sacroiliitis, and 14 (64%) had bilateral sacroiliitis. Of the 22 patients with abnormal scans, 20 had normal radiographs.[11]

EVALUATION AND MANAGEMENT

To be valid, a test must be an appropriate, purposeful procedure to demonstrate how and to what degree a lesion or dysfunction varies from normal. Heretofore the function of the lumbosacroiliac complex has not been thoroughly understood. Most current movement tests are inappropriate or misinterpreted, because even after an extensive work-up 85% of patients cannot be given a definitive diagnosis.[25] Ignorance of the cause of acute low back pain is so profound and pervasive that recent guidelines recommend no special interventions or diagnostic tests within the first month of symptoms for over 95% of patients.[1] Dysfunction of the sacroiliac joint is seldom included in evaluation procedures, and the majority of tests currently used do not reveal the problem when it exists.

Passive Straight-Leg Raising Test

The passive straight-leg raising test (PSLR) may be quite helpful in the differential evaluation of dysfunction of the sacroiliac joint, but it is more frequently interpreted in relation to nerve root pain and possible disk involvement,[40] even though false-positive and false-negative results are common.[38,41] A disk lesion is not the necessary cause of pain with PSLR; even if present, it may have nothing to do with pain other than possibly making it worse.[22]

The effects of the PSLR on dysfunction of the sacroiliac joints, although considerable, are not usually considered. Bohannon, Gajdosik, and LeVeau found a constant relationship between PSLR, pelvic rotation, and pelvic angle.[2] Pelvic rotation occurred in every subject by 9° of PSLR and usually before 4°.[2] Any dysfunction restriction in pelvic rotation may affect the PSLR test. Dysfunction of the sacroiliac joints also may cause a hamstring strain[8] or sciatic pain.[23]

The pull of the hamstrings on the ischial tuberosity with PSLR causes a force in posterior rotation that may ease the pain of an anterior dysfunction of the sacroiliac joints.[13,14] Mennell noted that as the ipsilateral innominate bone moves posteriorly with PSLR, the sacrum is carried posteriorly on the contralateral innominate bone; contralateral pain in the low back indicates an anterior dysfunction of the sacroiliac joint on the contralateral side.[28] Self-bracing is increased on the ipsilateral side with PSLR and released on the contralateral side. If at the conclusion of the PSLR test, the patient attempts to assist the examiner and actively holds back or lowers the leg with the hip flexors, ipsilateral pain in the low back may be increased. The eccentric contraction of the iliacus tends to pull the ipsilateral innominate bone anteriorly on the sacrum, increasing the pain of anterior dysfunction. Two tests help to confirm the sacroiliac joints as the most likely location of this pain:

1. If the patient stabilizes the anterior pelvis with the abdominal muscles by raising the head and shoulders and is then able to lower the leg without discomfort, the fault is in the sacroiliac joint and not the iliacus.

2. If the abdominal muscles are weak and cannot support the anterior pelvis, the patient should actively lower the leg against resistance applied by the examiner, using the hip extensors. The resultant force in posterior rotation eases the pain of anterior dysfunction. Ipsilateral pain in the low back with PSLR indicates anterior cephalic shearing of the innominate, which may compromise anterior dysfunction (see Figs. 12 and 13).

Thus, when performing the PSLR test, one must ask the patient whether the test causes or eases pain in the ipsilateral low back, whether it causes pain in the back on the contralateral side or down the ipsilateral leg, and whether the pain is deep between the hamstrings or in the biceps femoris and peroneus longus.

Confirmation and Correction

Given the complexities of the functional biomechanics of the sacroiliac joints, the considerable number and variety of affected tissues, changes in leg length and

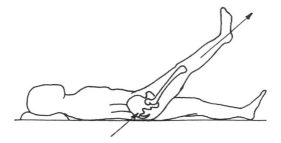

FIGURE 14.   Pulling on the leg in the long axis in hip flexion corrects the dysfunction and causes the leg to become shorter. Repeat at least three times with each leg, alternating. Check the leg length each time. (From DonTigny RL: Mechanics and treatment of the sacroiliac joint. J Man Manip Ther 1:3–12, 1993; with permission.)

gait, and apparent mimicking of the herniated intervertebral disk, it is hard to believe that the underlying cause is a subtle movement of the innominate bones on the sacrum. If the cause of so much low back pain is so simple, relief and management also should be simple—and they are! Although initial evaluation must include screening to eliminate potentially dangerous underlying conditions, manual correction of the sacroiliac joint to the self-bracing position is the simple procedure that provides essentially immediate relief to over 90% of all patients with low back pain.

Because the leg appears to lengthen when the anterosuperior iliac spine moves downward and the posterosuperior iliac spine moves upward as the innominate rotates anteriorly on the sacrum on an acetabular axis, it can be expected to appear shorter when the innominate is rotated upward anteriorly and downward posteriorly to the self-bracing position. The key phrase is "downward posteriorly," because fixation appears to occur in this position. The apparent shortening of the leg is a measurable, objective, positive, and predictable sign of correction, associated with relief of pain and restoration of function to the sacroiliac joint. The apparent shortening occurs with correction of unilateral dysfunction, when the long leg is on the painful side; with bilateral dysfunction, when both legs appear to be of equal length; with bilateral oblique dysfunction, when both sides are anterior, one more than the other; and with compromised bilateral dysfunction, when the apparently short leg is on the more painful side. This apparent change in leg length is accompanied by movement of the posterosuperior iliac spine caudad and medially on the sacrum. The difference in leg length does not cause dysfunction in the sacroiliac joints; rather, the dysfunction causes the changes in leg length. Because this dysfunction is easily corrected with mobilization, heel lifts are unnecessary.[15]

The test to correct and confirm anterior dysfunction is performed with the patient supine on a plinth. The examiner stands at the foot of the plinth, grasps each ankle, approximates the malleoli in the midline, and notes the comparative length of each leg. The relative position of each medial malleolus is an extension of the position of each ipsilateral acetabulum and indicates the position of the acetabulum relative to the sacrum.

Probably the simplest and safest method of mobilization to the self-bracing position is to grasp an ankle with both hands, to lift the leg to about 40° of PSLR, and to apply a strong sustained pull on the leg in the long axis for about 5–10 seconds (Fig. 14). No jerking, popping, or twisting is necessary. The examiner than puts the leg down and examines the relative length at the malleoli. The leg now appears to be

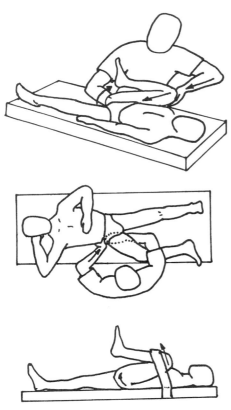

FIGURE 15. Sacroiliac dysfunction can be corrected and self-bracing restored by mobilizing the innominate bones posteriorly and downward on the sacrum by using the leg as a lever (top), by grasping the innominate directly and rotating (middle), or by using a strong isometric hip extension against a strap. (From DonTigny RL: Mechanics and treatment of the sacroiliac joint. J Man Manip Ther 1:3–12, 1993; with permission.)

shorter than before. The procedure then is repeated with the other leg, which also appears to shorten when measured from the navel to the distal aspect of the medial malleolus. When the procedure is repeated with the first leg, it probably will appear to shorten even more. The procedure is repeated with alternating legs until no more shortening occurs. The legs should be of equal length after correction. Because the sacroiliac joints are high-friction joints, they must be wobbled back into self-bracing a little bit at a time.

Other methods may be used to rotate the innominate bones posteriorly on the sacrum: (1) direct rotation of the innominate bone, using the leg as a lever, or (2)

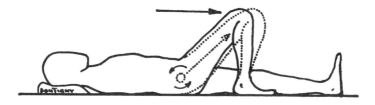

FIGURE 16. Active extension of the hip to project the knee distally and to rock the pelvis posteriorly is effective in restoring self-bracing. Alternate this exercise with each leg several times and repeat as necessary throughout the day. (From DonTigny RL: Function of the lumbosacroiliac complex as self-compensating force couple with a variable, force-dependent transverse axis: A theoretical analysis. J Man Manip Ther 2:87–93, 1994; with permission.)

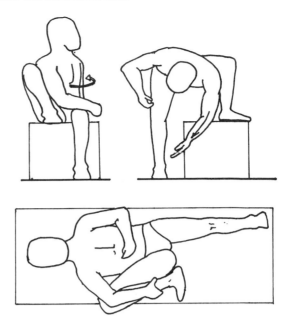

FIGURE 17. The patient should correct the dysfunction many times during the day with direct stretch while either sitting, standing, or lying. After the acute phase, correction should be done only when necessary. (From DonTigny RL: Mechanics and treatment of the sacroiliac joint. J Man Manip Ther 1:3–12, 1993; with permission.)

strong isometric hip extension (Fig. 15). The apparent leg length at the malleoli should be reexamined after each procedure. Occasionally the dysfunction may be so tight that it does not release with the first attempt at correction. In such cases, the physician corrects the other leg and then returns to the first leg, which will release much more easily. It is interesting and enlightening to mobilize or pull on a short or long leg and watch it become shorter.

Corrective Exercises

The patient must begin self-mobilization exercises as soon as possible after onset of symptoms to correct the dysfunction. In the simplest and most effective exercise, the patient lies supine with one hip and knee flexed so that the heel is as close as comfortably possible to the hip, then actively extends the hip, projecting the knee distally (Fig. 16). This exercise tilts the pelvis cephalad anteriorly and puts a little traction on the innominate bone, pulling it caudad posteriorly. The patient holds this position for 4 or 5 seconds, then relaxes and repeats the exercise with the other leg. The exercise is repeated at least 3 times with each leg.

A wide variety of exercises can be performed to accomplish the same result, including a direct stretch (Fig. 17) and a strong isometric hip extension (Fig. 18). Any of these exercises may be used, depending on individual response. The selected exercises should be performed alternately on each side at least 3 times and repeated many times throughout the day. Self-correction at bedtime allows the joints to stay relatively unstressed for several hours.

Onset or recurrence of dysfunction is prevented by active support of the anterior pelvis to maintain the self-bracing mechanism when the patient is standing, especially before leaning forward (Fig. 19). Depending on individual fitness, the muscles most involved in maintaining the self-bracing mechanism, including the abdominal musculature, gluteus maximus, and hamstrings may have to be strengthened.

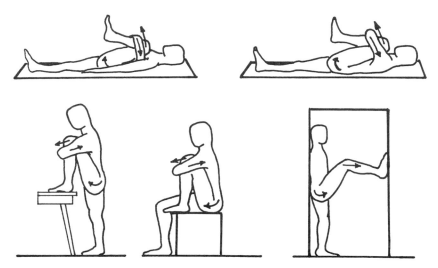

FIGURE 18. The patient may also use a strong isometric hip extension in any convenient position, alternating at least three times on each side. (From DonTigny RL: Mechanics and treatment of the sacroiliac joint. J Man Manip Ther 1:3–12, 1993; with permission.)

A good lumbosacral support may help to stabilize the unstable joint, but it should be put on when the patient is supine and after correction has been made. If the support is put on without correcting the dysfunction, it may increase pain by increasing pressure on the uncorrected sacroiliac joints. The support may be worn not only during the day to stabilize the pelvis, but also during sleep when the muscles and ligaments are at rest and the pelvis is less stable.

Patients may sleep comfortably in a supine position with a pillow under the upper thighs; lying on the side with the hips and knees flexed and a pillow between

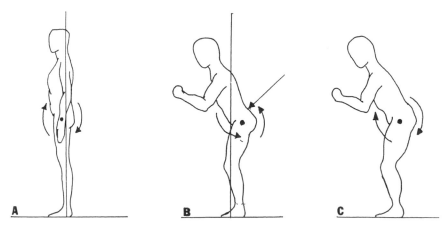

FIGURE 19. *A*, standing with a posterior pelvic tilt maintains self-bracing. *B*, dysfunction occurs with anterior rotation and loss of self-bracing. *C*, dysfunction can be prevented by maintaining self-bracing with support of the anterior pelvis by the abdominal muscles while the patient is leaning forward. (From DonTigny RL: Mechanics and treatment of the sacroiliac joint. J Man Manip Ther 1:3–12, 1993; with permission.)

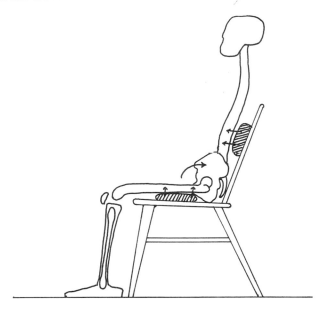

FIGURE 20.   Use of appropriate support maintains self-bracing while the patient is seated. (From DonTigny RL: Mechanics and treatment of the sacroiliac joint. J Man Manip Ther 1:3–12, 1993; with permission.)

the knees; or prone with the hip and knee of the painful side well-flexed. Silk or acetate pajamas decrease torsional pelvic stress when the patient turns in bed by decreasing friction with the sheets.

Pain on sitting can be minimized by placing a pad about 40 cm long by 20 cm wide by 3–4 cm thick under the upper thighs, just anterior to the ischial tuberosities. The pad unweights the ischial tuberosities and relieves ischemic pain by shunting the weight to the femoral heads, restoring some buttressing and exerting a posterior rotational force on the innominate bones to restore self-bracing. If a lumbar pad is used, it should be placed higher than the ilia to stabilize the vertebrae anteriorly and to avoid interference with the corrective posterior rotation of the innominate bones (Fig. 20). If a lumbar pad is used without the seat pad and placed too low, it may cause the innominate bones to rotate anteriorly, decreasing self-bracing and increasing pain.[15]

The importance of good posture cannot be overemphasized. A forward head posture allows the chest to flatten, thus decreasing anterior pelvic support and self-bracing. The anteriorly inclined pelvis impairs the hip flexor mechanism, leading to ambulation with an externally rotated thigh and substitution of hip adduction for hip flexion. This posture leads to a valgus deformity of the knee, improper patellar tracking, flattening of the longitudinal arch, and rolling over the hallux with eventual hallux valgus. The anteriorly inclined pelvis also may impair venous return from the lower extremities, increasing back pressure in the veins and leading to varicosities.

Modalities

Modalities are not helpful in the treatment of low back pain if the self-bracing mechanism remains impaired; however, after manual correction to the self-bracing position, modalities may provide a great deal of relief. A heating pad may be placed under the supine patient with electrical stimulator pads over the heating pad and under the posterosuperior and posteroinferior iliac spines. Stimulation is applied to comfortable tolerance. The pads are left in place for 30 minutes. My choice of current is 20–70 Hz biphasic stimulation, pyramidal at 10–30 seconds on cycle and 5–10 seconds off cycle. Subsequent massage decreases swelling and congestion in the gluteals. Electric stimulation may be applied to the biceps femoris and peroneus longus if they are sore. The patient is usually free of pain or at least much relieved after treatment.

Invasive Procedures

Norman and May treated over 300 patients with injection of local anesthetic into the sacroiliac joints. Relief of pain was immediate in patients who had both sensory changes and an absent Achilles reflex.[31] Therapeutic results were obtained by adding hydrocortisone to the anesthetic. Several patients with continuing low back pain after one or two laminectomies for the removal of disks were successfully treated by three or four injections.[31] Ray reported significant relief from idiopathic low back pain through the use of facet nerve blocks and sacroiliac desensitization with needle rhizotomies.[33] In a double-blind study, Ongley and associates successfully treated chronic low back pain accompanied by ligamentous insufficiency with manipulation of the sacroiliac joints, flexion exercises, and sclerosant injections into the adjacent ligaments.[32] Special attention should be paid to the tissue in the immediate vicinity of the posteroinferior iliac spine and to the superficial long posterior sacroiliac ligament.

Excellent relief of pain in the unstable sacroiliac joint has been reported after arthrodesis,[10,37] although this procedure totally prevents normal function and may have an adverse effect on the other pelvic structures. One researcher reported failures of the pubic symphysis in several patients after fusion of the sacroiliac joints; further surgery was required.[10] If fusion is considered, it may be advantageous to fuse in the self-bracing position.

CONCLUSION

The lumbosacroiliac complex appears to function as a self-compensating force-couple that generates a variable, force-dependent transverse axis, usually through the posterior aspect of the sacroiliac joint. This force-couple increases joint stability through a principle of self-bracing that allows greater ligamentous tension for the storage and release of energy and serves to balance forces of gravity, weight-loading, inertia, rotation, acceleration, and deceleration. Dysfunction may occur with anterior displacement of the line of gravity if anterior pelvic support fails to maintain self-bracing and friction. The resulting lesion, which may mimic disk dysfunction or give the impression of a multifactorial etiology, prevents normal function of the force-couple.

REFERENCES

1. Acute Low Back Problems in Adults. Clinical Practice Guideline No. 14. Rockville, MD, US Dept. of Health and Human Services, Agency for Health Care Policy and Research, 1994. AHCPR publication 95-0642.
2. Bohannon RW, Gajdosik R, LeVeau BF: Contribution of pelvic and lower limb motion to increases in the angle of passive straight leg raising. Phys Ther 65:474–476, 1985.
3. Bourdillon JF: Spinal Manipulation. 3rd ed. London, William Heinemann Medical Books, 1982.
4. Braddock GTF, quoted in Grieve GP: Common Vertebral Joint Problems. New York, Churchill Livingstone, 1981, pp 502–505.

5. Brook R: The sacroiliac joint. J Anat 58:299–305, 1924.
6. Brown T, Hansen RJ, Yorra AJ: Some mechanical tests on the lumbosacral spine with particular reference to the intervertebral discs. J Bone Joint Surg 39A:1135–1164, 1957.
7. Calguneri M, Bird HA, Wright V: Changes in joint laxity occurring during pregnancy. Ann Rheum Dis 41:126–128, 1982.
8. Cibulka MT, Rose SJ, Delitto A, et al: Hamstring muscle strain treated by mobilizing the sacroiliac joint. Phys Ther 66:1220–1223, 1986.
9. Colachis SC, Worden RE, Bechtol CO, et al: Movement of the sacroiliac joint in the adult male: A preliminary report. Arch Phys Med Rehabil 44:490–498, 1963.
10. Coventry MG, Trapper BM: Pelvic instability. J Bone Joint Surg 54A:83–101, 1972.
11. Davis P, Lentle BC: Evidence for sacroiliac disease as a common cause of low backache in women. Lancet 2:496–497, 1978.
12. Dihlman W: Diagnostic Radiology for the Sacroiliac Joints. Chicago, Year Book, 1980.
13. DonTigny RL: Function and pathomechanics of the sacroiliac joint. A review. Phys Ther 65:35–44, 1985.
14. DonTigny RL: Anterior dysfunction of the sacroiliac joint as a major factor in the etiology of idiopathic low back pain syndrome. Phys Ther 70:250–265, 1990.
15. DonTigny RL: Mechanics and treatment of the sacroiliac joint. J Man Manip Ther 1:3–12, 1993.
16. DonTigny RL: Measuring PSIS movement. Clin Manage 10:43–44, 1990.
17. DonTigny RL: Function of the lumbosacroiliac complex as self-compensating force couple with a variable, force-dependent transverse axis: A theoretical analysis. J Man Manip Ther 2:87–93, 1994.
18. Dorman TA: The Human Pelvis and the Use of Prolotherapy. San Luis Obispo, CA, Thomas A. Dorman, 1994.
19. Farfan HF, Cossette JW, Robertson GH, et al: The effects of torsion in the production of disc degeneration. J Bone Joint Surg 52A:468–497, 1970.
20. Farfan HF: Mechanical Disorders of the Low Back. Philadelphia, Lea & Febiger, 1973.
21. Grieve GP: The sacro-iliac joint. Physiotherapy 62:374, 1976.
22. Grieve GP: Common Vertebral Joint Problems. New York, Churchill Livingstone, 1981.
23. Hiltz DL: The sacroiliac joint as a source of sciatica: A case report. Phys Ther 56:1373, 1976.
24. Jayson M: Structure and function of the human spine. In Conference Proceedings: Engineering Aspects of the Spine. London, Mechanical Engineering Publications, 1980.
25. Kelsey JL: Idoopathic low back pain: Magnitude of the problem. In White AA, Gordon SL (eds): American Academy of Surgeons Symposium on Idiopathic Low Back Pain. St. Louis, Mosby, 1982.
26. Linton SJ, Kamwendo K: Low back schools. A critical review. Phys Ther 67:1375–1383, 1987.
27. McKenzie RA: The Lumbar Spine: Mechanical Diagnosis and Therapy. Waikanae, New Zealand, Spinal Publications Ltd., 1981.
28. Mennell JB: The Science and Art of Joint Manipulation: The Spinal Column. Vol. 2. London, J&A Churchill, 1952.
29. Nachemson AL: The lumbar spine: An orthopaedic challenge. Spine 1:59–71, 1976.
30. Norman GR: Sacroiliac disease and its relationship to lower abdominal pain. Am J Surg 116:54–56, 1968.
31. Norman GF, May A: Sacroiliac conditions simulating intervertebral disk syndrome. West J Surg Obstet Gynecol 64:461–462, 1956.
32. Ongley MJ, Klein RG, Dorman TA, et al: A new approach to the treatment of chronic low back pain. Lancet 2:143–146, 1987.
33. Ray CE: Percutaneous Radio-frequency Facet Nerve Blocks: Treatment of the Mechanical Low-back Syndrome. Burlington, MA, Radionics, 1982.
34. Roaf R: A study of the mechanics of spinal injuries. J Bone Joint Surg 42B:810–823, 1960.
35. Shah JS, Hampson WGJ, Jayson MIV: The distribution of surface strain in the cadaveric lumbar spine. J Bone Joint Surg 60B:246–251, 1978.
36. Shaw JT: The role of the sacroiliac joint as a cause of low back pain and dysfunction. In Vleeming A, Mooney V, Snijders C, Dorman T (eds): First Interdisciplinary World Congress on Low Back Pain and Its Relation to the Sacroiliac Joint. Rotterdam, ECO, 1992, pp 67–80.
37. Smith-Peterson MN: Arthrodesis of the sacroiliac joint. A new method of approach. J Orthop Surg 3:400–405, 1938.
38. Spangfort EV: The lumbar disc herniation. Acta Orthop Scand Suppl 142:5–95, 1972.
39. Thorstensson A, Nilsson J, Carlson H, Zomlefer MR: Trunk movements in human locomotion. Acta Physiol Scand 121:9–22, 1984.
40. Urban LM: The straight-leg-raising test: A review. J Orthop Sports Phys Ther 2:117–133, 1981.

41. Vaz M, Wadia RS, Gokhole SD: Another cause of positive crossed-straight leg raising test. N Engl J Med 299:779–780, 1978.
42. Vleeming A: Personal communication, 1993.
43. Vleeming A: Personal communication, 1994.
44. White AA, Panjabi M: Clinical Biomechanics of the Spine. Philadelphia, JB Lippincott, 1978.
45. White AA: Introduction. In White AA, Gordon SL (eds): American Academy of Surgeons Symposium on Idiopathic Low Back Pain. St. Louis, Mosby, 1982.
46. Wilson JC Jr: Low back pain and sciatica: A plea for better care of the patient. JAMA 200:705–712, 1967.

THOMAS A. DORMAN, MD

REFURBISHING LIGAMENTS WITH PROLOTHERAPY

Private Practice
San Luis Obispo, California

It is often said in modern medical circles that decay begins with birth, and this comment is not facetious. Contemporary medicine largely deals with degenerative disease, and the contemporary emphasis on arresting the degenerative processes is indeed not displaced. Antihypertensives, antihyperlipoproteinemics, antithrombotics, antiarthritics, and antiinflammatories, let alone antibiotics and antimalignant chemotherapy, are all modern pharmacologic approaches to disease. They are all predicated on the paradigm of retarding the inevitable decay of aging, of degeneration. Philosophically, this perspective is in tune with the Second Law of Thermodynamics, with *entropy*. The sun and solar system are in a decay curve. All we can do during our lives is retard the deterioration and make the best of the resources available. Entropy is a pessimistic world view. Philosophy governs life. We sometimes refer to philosophy with the terms *ideas, science* or *concepts*. The overriding dominance of entropy has not always characterized scientific thought. By this framework, the father of modern philosophy, Aristotle, was an optimist. Aristotle declared that life is an essential part of the universe and that life—by definition, growth of plants with the formation of new organic material, photosynthesis, and the cycle of birth and growth of the animal kingdom, the blossoming of species, and the process of evolution of each on our planet—are all *antientropic* incarnations. If Aristotle was right that life, the biosphere, is an essential part of the universe, then growth and life are natural. This philosophical introduction is necessary in anticipation of the following discus-

SPINE: State of the Art Reviews—Vol. 9, No. 2, May 1995
Philadelphia, Hanley & Belfus, Inc.

509

sion of prolotherapy because the pessimistic point of view has prevailed in contemporary scientific medicine and has represented a psychological bar to the acceptance of this concept.

PROLOTHERAPY

From the inception of the science of pathology, cycles of tissue reaction to disease and injury have been recognized; they are the essentials of the discipline. Early pathologists described red hepatization followed by gray hepatization and, finally, healing in the case of lobar pneumococcal pneumonia. The description of the injurious process in the connective tissue and its repair has not been neglected, but since the process is simple histologically, it has not been subject to much repeated research or analysis. The inflammation that precedes and initiates the repair process of connective tissue was first described by Eli Mechnikoff[10] and more detailed descriptions of the dynamic process elaborated by Cohnheim,[2] who studied the process microscopically in the living capillaries of rabbit ears. Modern pathologic preparations of both dead and fixed histology allows study of an imaged representation of a moment in time, and only through serial histologic studies of parallel situations can we approximate an understanding of the *dynamic process*. Nonetheless, enough information is available from a combination of these methods to state that healing in connective tissues is a dynamic process initiated by the injury, and, through a combination of the humoral agents of inflammation liberated by the cells at the site of the injury and an interaction with the mesenchymal migrant cells, both from the hemopoietic system and of mesenchymal origin such as fibroblasts, initiate the *cascade of healing*. What is the endpoint of healing? It depends on variables, including the following:

1. The extent and severity of the injury
2. Whether the damage is permanent or repairable
3. The nature of the injured tissue (some tissues respond differently)
4. The strength of the healing stimulus
5. The duration of healing

An extraordinary observation of the healing process in almost all tissues is the phenomenon of *cessation of healing*. Experiments have shown that after resection of half a liver in dogs, the remaining tissue grows appropriately to the right size, mass, and biochemical capacity. Regeneration then ceases. The *servomechanism* by which the intact organism regulates the termination of the healing process is unknown. Cessation of healing is a subcategory of the more general issue of *morphogenetics*. The whole process of maintenance of size and form appropriate to the age, size, and biochemical requirements of organs remains an enigma in contemporary biologic sciences, an enigma marked by the extraordinary absence of discussion of the problem in scientific circles.

The process of inflammation initiates repair following injury in the mesenchym. Connective tissue—collagenous tissue such as ligaments, fasciae and tendon—is known to be subject to repair through the same mechanism. The repair process of these ligamentous fascial structures is at times deficient or incomplete. The terms *deficient* and *incomplete* are relative in the sense that clinical experience has shown that enhancement of the repair process yields superior clinical results and it is *assumed* in orthopedic medical circles that the natural healing process following the injury was inadequate, that it was *abnormal*. The phenomenon of the provocation of *hypertrophy* of collagenous ligamentous, fascial, and tendinous tissue has been confirmed. Prolotherapy is the provocation of the laying down of increased amounts of *normal* collagenous material in ligament, tendon, or fascia, which enhances the function of these tissues at the site concerned. The process is achieved by relighting: provoking inflammation at the site.

Scars—Good and Bad Healing

Scar tissue has a number of *mechanical* properties that differ from those of normal connective tissue that are considered disadvantageous. Scars can be recognized histologically as different from normal connective tissue. George Hackett, one of the first practitioners of prolotherapy, realized that in situations where ligaments are *relaxed* (his term for ligament insufficiency), hypertrophy of the ligament represented an advantage; in contrast, scar formation would be a disadvantage. Was there any prospect of achieving ligamentous hypertrophy without scar? In setting out a therapeutic "road map," Hackett apparently envisioned that the injections should:

1. Be effective
2. Provoke as little pain as feasible
3. Be safe
4. Be easy to learn and perform
5. Require the minimal number of repetitions
6. Work generically, i.e., be effective in as many people as possible
7. Yield hypertrophy of normal tissue
8. Avoid scarring

Following this road map, a series of informal empiric trials evolved in the 1940s and 1950s, first in animals and later in patients with injured ligaments, in the use of a number of sclerosing agents that by this point Hackett had renamed *proliferant agents*. It was determined that benefit could be achieved clinically by the use of a modicum of polypharmacy. The chief proliferant agents used today, as judged by the frequency of usage, are glucose, glycerin, and phenol. They are usually used in the following combination: phenol 1.25%, glucose 12.5%, glycerin 12.5%, prepared with 0.5% of lidocaine for local analgesia in water. This preparation is also called P25G or P2G.

Klein[1] and Banks[8] have classified the injectable proliferating solutions that initiate the wound healing cascade into the following categories:

1. Irritants, which cause a direct chemical tissue injury and attract granulocytes. Phenol, quinine, and tannic acid are agents in this category.

2. Osmotic shock agents, which cause bursting of cell membranes leading to local tissue damage. Hyperosmolar dextrose (12.5 to 15% maximum) and glycerin are the most common examples.

3. Chemotactic agents, which activate the inflammatory cascade. Sodium morrhuate is a prototype of this group. These compounds are the direct biosynthetic precursors of the mediators of inflammation, i.e., prostaglandins, leukotrienes, and thromboxanes.

4. Particulates, such as pumice flour, which are small particles of about 1 µ. They lead to longer-lasting irritation and the attraction of macrophages to the site.

Evidence of Proliferant Effect

Extensive literature exists that documents the histologic scar formation in the mode of sclerotherapy.[15] Although this old research has not been confirmed in the contemporary scientific mode, pathologists report scar formation from time to time in biopsies obtained in routine surgical and medical practice. This subject is considered as accepted general knowledge. Therefore, research in the context of the use of proliferant therapy needs to be seen as an addition to the established body of knowledge regarding the healing of connective tissue. George Hackett reported in the 1950s on the histologic changes of the tendo Achilles of rats treated with proliferant therapy. These were open studies and were considered entirely satisfactory proof of the proliferant effect in the limited circles that had adopted these techniques, the Sclerotherapy Society, and were ignored by the rest of the medical establishment. The next landmark in the study of prolotherapy was a blinded animal study combining histology, electron microscopy, and mechanical evaluation of rabbit ligaments. King Liu et al.[7] used sodium morrhuate in the medial collateral ligaments of rabbit knees and published their findings in 1982. The histologic and mechanical beneficial effects of proliferant therapy in this experimental model were established categorically. The remaining, and minor, question of a parallel phenomenon on human tissue was established with the taking of biopsies of posterior sacroiliac ligaments, which were performed before and after treatment in three patients with chronic low back pain.[9] Treatment consisted of a series of six weekly injections into lumbar and sacroiliac ligaments, fascia, and facet capsular sites using a connective tissue proliferant (dextrose-glycerine-phenol) combined with mobilization and flexion/extension exercises. Biopsies performed 3 months after completion of injections demonstrated fibroblastic hyperplasia on light microscopy and increases in average ligament diameter on electronmicroscopy from a pretreatment of .055 ± 0.26 μm to .087 ± .041 μm posttreatment ($p < 0.001$). Range of motion significantly improved posttreatment in rotation ($p < 0.001$), flexion ($p < 0.015$), and side flexion ($p < 0.001$), as did visual analogue pain ($p < 0.001$) and disability ($p < 0.001$) scores. Figure 1 illustrates the histology of human ligaments before and after prolotherapy. Figure 2 shows electron micrographs of the same samples.

Mechanics and Ligament Proliferation

Accepting that prolotherapy provokes hyperplasia of ligament tissue, an increased amount of collagen, and the absence of damage as far as can be judged histologically, an assessment was needed regarding the mechanical effect of prolotherapy in human ligaments to match the mechanical observations made by King Liu. This issue was addressed through the treatment of the joint capsule and injured ligaments of the knees of athletes. The study was conducted over 9 months in a private orthopedic office. Thirty patients with knee pain were seen during the enrollment period, but in only five knees in four patients was it possible to obtain recordings after treatment. All of the participants had substantial ligament instability. All measurements were taken by one researcher. The patients underwent multiple injections and underwent repeat measurements within 9 months. Subjective symptoms were obtained at entry and exit from the study. Ligament stability was measured by a commercially available computerized instrument that measures ligament function objectively and reliably in a complete three-dimensional format.[11,14] It consists of a chair equipped with a six-component force platform and a six-degree freedom electrogoniometer. With computer integrated force and motion measurements, a standardized series of clinical laxity tests can be performed and an objective report obtained. Prior studies have compared clinical testing with objective tests[3] and have established reproducibility.[5] The proliferant solution used in these cases was P25G.

The proliferant injections were "peppered" into the lax ligaments usually at 2-week intervals, with each ligament being treated an average of four times. Between 30 mL and 40 mL of the proliferant solution was injected into the appropri-

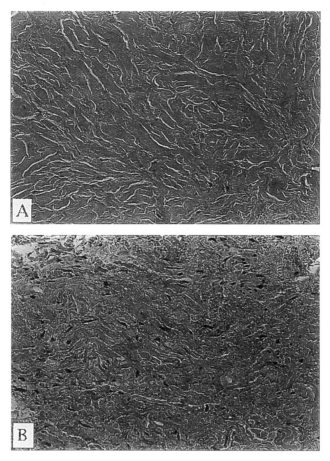

FIGURE 1. An H & E stain shows the histology of human ligaments before (*A*) and after (*B*) prolotherapy.

ate portion of the joint ligaments. Details regarding the injection technique are published elsewhere.[12]

Table 1 summarizes the findings of the five knees in the three-dimensional computerized format. No systemic or general complications occurred in any of the cases.

Wolff's Law

It has been established since the turn of the last century that the musculoskeletal systems of mammals respond to the lines of force through reinforcement. This has been called Wolff's Law after the scientist who described the lines of force in bony trabeculae first. This observation of the nature of healing in mesenchymal tissues in the presence of forces and movement is largely the basis on which modern early mobilization after disease and the use of exercises and mobilization in rehabilitation and physiotherapy has gained its reputation. The use of exercises and mobilization in orthopedic medicine is no exception. Although the observation that *healing in the presence of movement* is an advantage with the use of prolotherapy, it has not been proved experimentally.

TABLE 1. Results of Prolotherapy in Five Knees*

Pt.	90°/0° Flx/Rtn		90°/10° IR Flx/Rtn		30°/0° Flx/Rtn		80° Int Rtn/Ext Rtn Stress in Deg	
Rx	Before	After	Before	After	Before	After	Before	After
DT27ML	10	6	6	3	12	5	38	33
R	9	8	6	3	20	13	47	36
GS35MR	13	8	8	4	10	7	37	37
SW31FR	7	5	7	1	5	2	54	41
KW43PR	8	4	7	3	5	0	40	31
p value	0.013		0.002		0.005		0.03	

* Objective and subjective data (all measurements in mm).
MCL = medial collateral ligament; LCL = lateral collateral ligament; PCL = posterior cruciate ligament; ACL = anterior cruciate ligament; caps = capsule

SUMMARY

The road map set out by Hackett has been achieved. The safety of the proliferant injections has been confirmed[4] and the mechanical and clinical outcome estab-

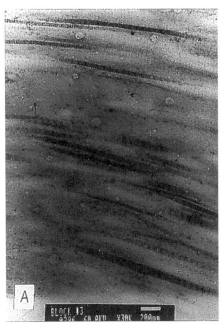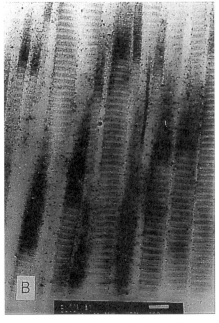

FIGURE 2. Electron micrographs of the samples seen in Figure 1 depicting the collagen of human ligaments before (A) and after (B) prolotherapy.

TABLE 1.   *(Cont.)*

Areas Treated	Subjective Before Treatment	Subjective After 9 Months Follow-up
MCL; LCL; PCL; ACL Med/lat caps	Pain; instability; unable to run, play tennis; feels insecure with left medial menisectomy 1982	No pain, more stable; able to run; starting to play tennis + less aware of knees
MCL; LCL; PCL; ACL; Med/lat caps	Right partial menisectomy 1984	
MCL; LCL; ACL; PCL Med caps	Sprained R knee skiing March 1986; knee unstable; weak; unable to bicycle	More stable; able to bicycle 30–40 miles
MCL; LCL; PCL; Med/lat./ant caps	Right medial menisectomy 1971; pain and minimal activity level	No pain; more stable; moderate to marked level of activities; able to cycle, waterski
MCL; LCL; PCL; Ant/post Med/lat caps	Right knee pain since February 1985 when she fell, causing fracture/dislocation and instability	Decrease in pain; more stable; tolerating increase in activities and starting resistive exercises

From Ongley MJ, Dorman TA, Eek BC, et al: Ligament instability of knees: A new approach to treatment. Man Med 3:152–154, 1988; with permission.

lished.[13] The technique of the injections of irritant material into connective tissue including ligaments, fasciae, and tendons is now known to provoke hyperplasia of normal connective tissue, which enhances the function of these tissues. These functions represent mechanical strength (binding) as well as the storage and release of elastic energy, enhancing the efficiency and the normal range of movement.

REFERENCES

1. Banks A: A rationale for prolotherapy. J Orthop Med 13:54–59, 1991.
2. Cohnheim JF: Lectures on General Pathology (English translation). New York, Dover Publications, 1968 (original, London, 1889).
3. Daniel DM, Malcolm LL, Losse G, et al: Instrument measurement of anterior laxity of the knee. J Bone Joint Surg 67A:720–725, 1985.
4. Dorman TA: Prolotherapy: A survey. J Orthop Med 15:2, 1993.
5. Highgenboten CL: The reliability of the Genucom knee analysis system. Presented at the Second European Congress of Knee Surgery and Arthroscopy, Basel, Switzerland, September 29, 1986.
6. Hippocrates: The Genuine Works of Hippocrates (Francis Adams, trans.). Baltimore, Williams & Wilkins, 1946.
7. King Liu Y, Tipton C, Matthews RD, et al: An in situ study of the influence of a sclerosing solution in rabbit medial collateral ligaments and its junction strength. Conn Tiss Res 11:95–102, 1983.
8. Klein: The Theory and Practice of Prolotherapy, 12th annual meeting of the American Association of Orthopaedic Medicine, Palm Springs, California, 1995.
9. Klein R, Dorman T, Johnson C: Prolotherapy in back pain. J Neurol Orthop Med Surg 10:123–126, 1989.
10. Metchnikoff E: Lectures on the Comparative Pathology of Inflammation. New York, Dover Publications, 1968 (original, 1893).
11. Oliver JH, Coughlin LP: An analysis of knee evaluation using clinical techniques and the Genucom knee analysis system. Presented at the interim meeting of the American Orthopedic Society for Sports Medicine. Las Vagas, January 23–24, 1985.
12. Ongley MJ, Dorman TA, Eek BC, et al: Ligament instability of knees: A new approach to treatment. Man Med 3:152–154, 1988.
13. Ongley MJ, Klein RG, Dorman TA et al: A new approach to the treatment of chronic back pain. Lancet 2:143–146, 1987.

14. Selsnick H, Oliver J, Virgin C: Analysis of knee ligament testing-Genucom and clinical exams. Presented at the annual meeting of the American Orthopedic Society for Sports Medicine, July 14–17, 1986, Sun Valley, Idaho.
15. Yeomans FC (ed): Sclerosing Therapy: The Injection Treatment of Hernia, Hydrocele, Varicose Veins and Hemorrhoids. Baltimore, William & Wilkins, 1939.

INDEX

Entries in **boldface type** indicate complete chapters.